CATECHOLAMINES

Physiology, Pharmacology, and Pathology for Students and Clinicians

CATECHOLAMINES

Physiology, Pharmacology, and Pathology
for Students and Clinicians

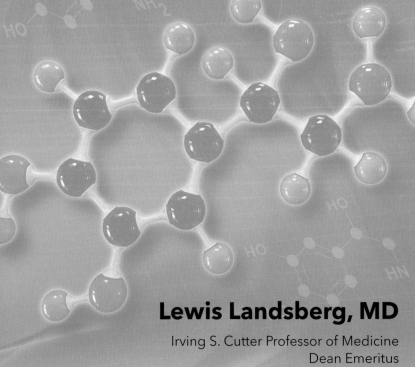

Lewis Landsberg, MD

Irving S. Cutter Professor of Medicine
Dean Emeritus
Director, Northwestern Comprehensive
Center on Obesity (NCCO)
Northwestern University Feinberg School of Medicine
Chicago, Illinois

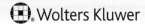. Wolters Kluwer

Philadelphia • Baltimore • New York • London
Buenos Aires • Hong Kong • Sydney • Tokyo

Executive Editor: Rebecca Gaertner
Senior Development Editor: Kristina Oberle
Production Project Manager: Marian Bellus
Marketing Manager: Rachel Mante Leung
Design Coordinator: Stephen Druding
Senior Manufacturing Coordinator: Beth Welsh
Prepress Vendor: S4Carlisle Publishing Services

9 8 7 6 5 4 3 2 1

Printed in China

Library of Congress Cataloging-in-Publication Data

ISBN-13: 978-1-4963-7531-5
ISBN-10: 1-4963-7531-9

Cataloging-in-Publication data available on request from the Publisher.

To the memory of Julius Axelrod

And to Jill, Alison, and Judd

Preface

E xperiments with extracts of adrenal glands in the late 19th century ushered in a hundred years of research on catecholamines and the sympathoadrenal system; these investigations ultimately provided the foundation of much basic biology that we take for granted today. The concepts of circulating hormones, neurochemical transmission, stimulus secretion coupling, second messengers, cell surface receptors, and G proteins all owe their origin to investigation of the sympathoadrenal system. The extraordinary number of Nobel Prizes awarded for work engendered by research on catecholamines bears witness to the unique and enduring scientific import of this area of medicine.

I have been thinking about catecholamines and the sympathoadrenal system for the past 50 years. I recall that my daughter, at age six, produced her first book that she called "catacolamines." It consisted of one sentence: "catacolamines are very complicated." She was right. My appreciation for the complexities and importance of these compounds has only grown over the years. My aim in writing this book is to address the complications and to share the insights I have gained with students who are learning about catecholamines and with clinicians whose daily activities involve pharmaceuticals that impact the function of the sympathoadrenal system in many different ways.

My interest in catecholamines began as a research associate in the laboratory of Julius Axelrod at the National Institutes of Health in the mid-1960s. It was an exciting period in the annals of catecholamine research, and Axelrod's laboratory was one of those at the forefront. He had managed to obtain tritiated norepinephrine (NE) for use as a biologic tracer in order to study the metabolic disposition and tissue distribution of NE after intravenous injection in laboratory rodents. These experiments led to a remarkable, and unexpected, finding: the tracer NE was rapidly cleared from the circulation but could be recovered, unchanged, from the tissues of injected rats hours later. Subsequent experiments demonstrated conclusively that the tracer NE was taken up into the sympathetic nerve terminals of innervated organs and stored with endogenous NE in the storage granules of the sympathetic nerves. There were several incredibly important implications of these experiments including: 1) the uptake process whereby NE is taken up in sympathetic nerve terminals was identified, and established as a major route of inactivation of NE; 2) compounds that blocked the uptake of catecholamines were identified, thus opening up a whole new class of pharmacologic agents; 3) uptake of the tracer NE into the sympathetic nerve terminals permitted the measurement of NE turnover rates in different tissues, a finding that ultimately enabled the assessment of sympathetic activity in different organ systems.

My contribution was recognizing the potential of NE turnover as a measure of sympathetic activity and the utilization of NE turnover as a direct and useful measure of organ-specific sympathetic outflow. At the time, there was no way to directly assess the activity of the sympathetic nervous system (SNS), a limitation that precluded appreciation of the role played by the SNS in the regulation of physiologic processes. The application of the NE turnover technique permitted, for the first time, characterization of the SNS responses in a variety of physiologic and pathophysiologic circumstances. My colleague James B. Young and I utilized these techniques to explore the SNS response in many situations relevant to clinical medicine.

It is impossible to understand normal physiology with an imperfect knowledge of autonomic function. Much of the altered physiology that characterizes common disease states reflects normal physiology gone awry. It is the purpose of this book to provide a comprehensive, clinically relevant, and authoritative summary of how catecholamines regulate bodily functions in health and in disease, and how this knowledge has spawned an extensive pharmacopeia of widely used drugs. As such, this book should be useful to medical and graduate students, and to clinicians, particularly internists, cardiologists, endocrinologists, intensivists, and anesthesiologists.

The book is divided into five parts with a bibliography following each: Part I: Fundamental aspects of catecholamine biology; Part II: Physiology of the sympathoadrenal system; Part III: Pathophysiology involving the sympathoadrenal system; Part IV: Pharmacology of the sympathoadrenal system; and Part V: Tumors of the sympathoadrenal system.

Lewis Landsberg
October 2016

Acknowledgments

I am indebted to Rebecca Gaertner at LWW for her encouragement and helpful suggestions as this book took shape. Thanks also to Kristina Oberle at LWW for her skillful help in formatting the manuscript.

Special thanks to Linda Carey for her indispensable help in producing the manuscript and developing the figures, and for her meticulous attention to detail throughout the production of this book. Special thanks also to Karen Kelley for outstanding help with information technology.

It is a pleasure to acknowledge my long-term colleague Dr. James B. Young for the major role he played in the experiments presented here and for the many thoughtful discussions we had about the functions of the sympathoadrenal system over the many years of our collaboration.

Contents

The Role of the Sympathoadrenal System in Physiologic Adaptation and the Pathophysiology of Disease States

Pharmacology

Tumors of the Sympathoadrenal System

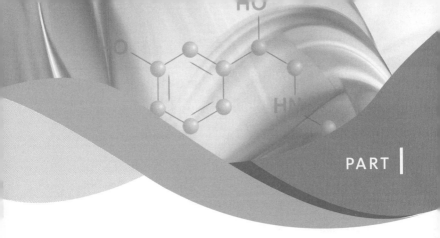

Fundamental Aspects of
Catecholamine Biology

Introduction: Overview of the Sympathoadrenal System

Epinephrine (E) was discovered in extracts of adrenal glands at the end of the 19th century and was reasonably well characterized shortly thereafter. It was thus the first hormone with a known chemical structure (Fig. 1.1). Over the ensuing century, catecholamine research resulted in many important discoveries that elucidated many fundamental biologic processes with wide applicability (Tables 1.1 and 1.2). These processes included neurochemical transmission, cell surface receptors, transmitter inactivation by reuptake, storage in subcellular granules, release by exocytosis, signal transduction and second messengers, G-proteins, and reversible protein phosphorylation in the activation and deactivation of enzymes and receptors. Nobel prizes have been awarded to 10 scientists for research involving catecholamines (Tables 1.1 and 1.2).

The overview provided in this chapter gives a general outline of the autonomic nervous system (ANS) and prepares the groundwork for appreciating the physiology and pharmacology detailed in subsequent sections.

The naturally occurring catecholamines

The naturally occurring, biologically important catecholamines are epinephrine (E), norepinephrine (NE), and dopamine (DA) (Table 1.3; Fig. 1.1). Present throughout the animal kingdom, catecholamines are found in protozoa and invertebrates, as well as vertebrates. In invertebrates, the predominant catecholamine is DA, which appears to serve as a neurotransmitter. In vertebrates, all three major

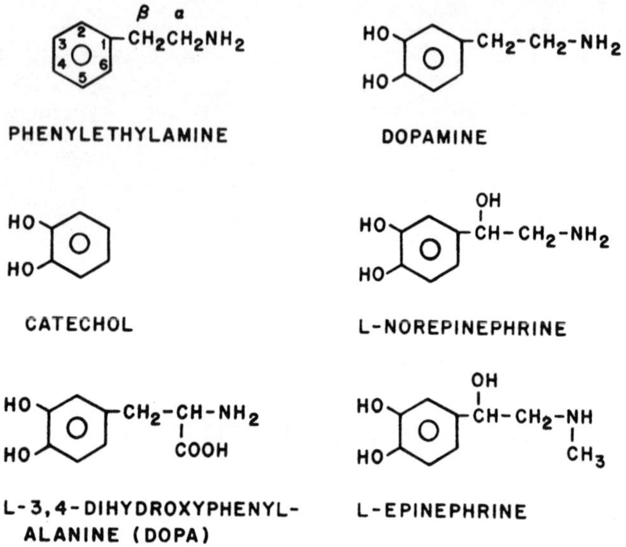

FIGURE 1.1. Structures of naturally occurring catecholamines and related compounds. The conventional numbering system for ring and side chain substituents is shown for phenylethylamine, which may be considered the parent compound of many sympathomimetic amines. Catecholamines are hydroxylated at positions 3 and 4 on the ring. (From Landsberg L, Young JB. Catecholamines and the adrenal medulla. In: Bondy PK, Rosenberg LE, eds. *Metabolic Control and Disease.* 8th ed. Philadelphia, PA: WB Saunders; 1980:1621–1693.)

catecholamines are found with variation in the relative proportions in the peripheral nerves and adrenal medulla. For example, in amphibians, E is the predominant adrenergic neurotransmitter in distinction to mammals that utilize NE at sympathetic neuroeffector junctions. In mammals, for practical purposes, E is limited to the central nervous system (CNS) and to chromaffin cells of the adrenal medulla. (The term "chromaffin" is a portmanteau word derived from chromium and affinity; chromaffin cells darken markedly on exposure to dilute solutions of chromium salts.) Catecholamines, therefore, are widely distributed in nature, phylogenetically ancient, and it may thus be inferred that they act as signaling molecules throughout the animal kingdom.

Embryology of the sympathoadrenal system

The sympathoadrenal (SA) system is derived from the neural crest. Early in embryonic development SA precursor cells migrate ventrally from the neuraxis and establish the sympathetic ganglia and the chromaffin cells of the adrenal medulla. The differentiation into sympathetic neurons and adrenal medullary chromaffin cells occurs after migration out of the neural crest but before the precursors

TABLE 1.1	**Landmark Discoveries in Catecholamine Research: Structure of First Circulating Hormone (Epinephrine); First Evidence for Both Neurochemical Transmission and for Specific Cell Surface Receptors; and Termination of Action by Uptake into the Sympathetic Nerve Endings**

- **Oliver and Shafer (1894)**
  - Adrenal extracts raise blood pressure
- **Abel (1897) and Takamine (1900)**
  - Isolated and purified active principle
  - Called epinephrine in U.S., adrenaline in U.K.
- **Stolz (1904) and Dakin (1905)**
  - Synthesized racemic adrenaline
  - First hormone with identified chemical structure
- **Lewandowsky (1899), Langley (1904), and Elliott (1904)**
  - Adrenal extracts mimic the effects of sympathetic nerve stimulation
  - The concept of neurochemical transmission is born
- **Barger and Dale[a] (1910)**
  - Structure activity relationships of "sympathomimetic amines"
  - Primary amines (like NE) more closely resemble sympathetic stimulation than secondary amines (like E)
- **Cannon (1921)**
  - Stimulation of sympathetic nerves releases an adrenaline-like substance
- **Von Euler[a] (1946)**
  - NE identified as the adrenergic neurotransmitter
- **Ahlquist (1948)**
  - Based on differential potencies for stimulatory and excitatory actions of sympathomimetic agonists the concept of distinct alpha and beta receptors is proposed
- **Axelrod[a] (1961)**
  - Identified NE uptake (and reuptake) into sympathetic nerve endings

[a]Denotes Nobel prize.
NE, norepinephrine; E, epinephrine.

destined to become chromaffin cells invade the anlagen of the developing adrenal cortex. Bone morphogenetic proteins derived from the dorsal aorta play a role in the differentiation of the neural crest cells into SA precursors. Nerve growth factor(s) derived from innervated tissues are involved in the development and maintenance of the sympathetic nervous system (SNS). Although the adrenal cortex is not required for the differentiation of adrenal medullary chromaffin cells, it is necessary for the synthesis of E, accomplished by the induction of the E-forming enzyme in the cytoplasm of chromaffin cells. In the sympathetic nerves innervating sweat glands, a phenotypic change in neurotransmitter from NE to acetylcholine (Ach) occurs during development, an example of the plasticity that exists in the developing nervous system.

TABLE 1.2	Landmark Discoveries in Catecholamine Research: Signal Transduction; Subcellular Storage and Release by Exocytosis; Second Messengers; G-proteins; Reversible Protein Phosphorylation in Receptor Desensitization and Enzyme Activation

- **Blaschko and Welch (1953), Hillarp (1953)**
  - Storage in subcellular organelles
- **Krebs[a] and Fischer (1955)**
  - Protein phosphorylation activates hepatic phosphorylase; inactivated by dephosphorylation
- **De Robertis and Vaz Ferreira (1957), Coupland (1965)**
  - Release by exocytosis
- **Sutherland[a] (1962)**
  - Catecholamine action through stimulation of adenylyl cyclase; cyclic AMP as second messenger; phosphodiesterase system metabolizes cyclic AMP
  - Eventually established (several groups) that cyclic AMP activated phosphorylation
- **Rodbell[a] (1972), Gilman[a] (1981)**
  - G-protein transducers between receptor activation and cellular effect
- **Murad[a] (1978)**
  - Inhibitory G proteins; cyclic GMP; nitrous oxide
- **Lefkowitz[a] and Kobilka[a] (1983)**
  - Beta adrenergic receptor coupled to G proteins; desensitization associated with beta receptor phosphorylation

[a]Denotes Nobel prize.
AMP, adenosine monophosphate.

TABLE 1.3	Biologically Important Catecholamines in Humans: Epinephrine, Norepinephrine, Dopamine

- **Epinephrine**
  - Circulating hormone of the adrenal medulla
  - Neurotransmitter within the CNS (brainstem)
- **Norepinephrine**
  - Neurotransmitter at peripheral sympathetic nerve endings
  - Neurotransmitter within the CNS
- **Dopamine**
  - Neurotransmitter within the CNS
  - Peripheral neurotransmitter in selected areas (small intensely fluorescent cells in sympathetic ganglia and in carotid body)
  - Autocrine or paracrine function (kidney, gut) after synthesis from circulating DOPA

CNS, central nervous system; DOPA, 3,4-dihydroxyphenylalanine.

The extra-adrenal chromaffin cells

As the SA precursor cells migrate ventrally from the neuraxis, some of these precursors destined to become chromaffin cells remain associated with the sympathetic neuronal precursors and form the extra-adrenal chromaffin cells. Aggregates of these cells are located in and around the preaortic plexuses, the largest of which is known as the organ of Zuckerkandl. These cells are prominent in fetal and neonatal life and tend to regress with aging. They store NE (not E) and are not innervated; their function is unknown, although they serve as a nidus for the subsequent development of extra-adrenal pheochromocytomas.

Central nervous system control of the sympathoadrenal system

The SNS and the adrenal medulla form a distinct unit that operates under direction of the CNS. Although the activity of these two components is always coordinated centrally to defend the constancy of the internal environment, the activity of the two systems varies widely in different physiologic circumstances; the adrenal medulla, for example, is frequently stimulated when the SNS is suppressed. The major factor responsible for the generation of catecholamine-mediated effects is the stimulatory output from the CNS centers that regulate the SA activity. Although the full physiologic expression of SA stimulation is modified by a variety of factors operating at the neuroeffector junctions, the level of central sympathetic outflow is the major determinant of the physiologic actions regulated by the SA system. Central SA outflow sets the gain; other factors fine-tune the responses. Autonomic reflexes do exist independent of descending central regulation but these are clinically important only after central connections are interrupted as in spinal cord injury.

CNS regulation of SA outflow has a number of important implications for the maintenance of homeostasis, but none more interesting or important than the integration of SA outflow with voluntary activity. CNS regulation permits anticipation of an event to initiate SNS-mediated changes in the circulation and metabolism before the actual event ("fight or flight" for example) takes place, thus limiting the impact on the internal milieu. In other words, the SA response can be anticipatory rather than merely reactive.

Structural organization of the autonomic nervous system

The ANS is comprised of two major divisions: the sympathetic and the parasympathetic. In distinction to the somatic nervous system, which controls the movement of the voluntary striated musculature, the ANS regulates involuntary or vegetative functions. Although useful for heuristic purposes, the distinction between somatic and autonomic is not complete as somatic activation is frequently accompanied by autonomic discharge. Some distinctions between the somatic nervous system and ANS are shown in Table 1.4.

In Figure 1.2, the overall anatomic organization of the SA system is shown; Figure 1.3 and Table 1.5 present the basic anatomy of the ANS in schematic form.

TABLE 1.4	Somatic and Autonomic Nervous Systems
Autonomic	**Somatic**
Unconscious	Conscious
Innervates smooth muscle and glands	Innervates striated muscle
Synapse in ganglia outside the CNS	Direct innervation from the CNS
Preganglionic fibers are myelinated; postganglionic are unmyelinated	Somatic nerves are myelinated
Ground plexus of terminal fibers in innervated tissues	Discrete motor endplates
Dispersion of central outflow at level of the ganglia	Discrete innervation of motor units
Representative functions: cardiac stimulation; vasomotor tone; glandular secretion; heat conservation and dissipation; visceral smooth muscle contraction	Function: voluntary movement

CNS, central nervous system.

Preganglionic neurons in the intermediolateral cell column of the spinal cord synapse with postganglionic sympathetic neurons in the sympathetic ganglia. Note that the adrenal medulla is analogous to the postganglionic sympathetic nerves; it receives a preganglionic cholinergic innervation from the splanchnic nerves and releases E into the circulation. Nerves that utilize Ach as their neurotransmitter are referred to as cholinergic; those utilizing NE are called adrenergic, per the suggestion of Sir Henry Dale in the 1930s (Table 1.6).

Intracellular storage of catecholamines in sympathetic nerve endings and chromaffin cells

After biosynthesis from tyrosine in sympathetic nerve endings and in adrenal medullary chromaffin cells, catecholamines are stored in discrete subcellular organelles referred to as "chromaffin granules" in the adrenal medulla and dense core vesicles in the sympathetic nerve endings. These organelles have many similarities and a few differences notably the larger size of the chromaffin granules (Figs. 1.4 and 1.5). They play a role in catecholamine biosynthesis and represent a large storage pool in which the catecholamines are protected from enzymatic degradation by monoamine oxidase (MAO).

General functions of the autonomic nervous system: steady state and "fight or flight"

Maintaining homeostasis is the overriding function of the ANS, a concept pioneered by Harvard physiologist Walter B. Cannon. Functioning below the conscious level, the ANS regulates bodily processes that maintain the constancy of the internal environment. The circulation, digestion, and metabolism, for

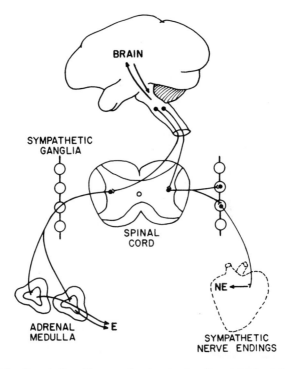

FIGURE 1.2. Organization of the sympathoadrenal system. Descending tracts from the medulla, pons, and hypothalamus synapse with preganglionic sympathetic neurons in the spinal cord, which in turn innervate the adrenal medulla directly or synapse in paravertebral ganglia with postganglionic sympathetic neurons. The latter give rise to sympathetic nerves, which are distributed widely to viscera and blood vessels. Release of E or NE at the adrenal medulla or at sympathetic nerve endings occurs in response to a downward flow of nerve impulses from regulatory centers in the brain. E, epinephrine; NE, norepinephrine. (From Landsberg L, Young JB. Catecholamines and the adrenal medulla. In: Bondy PK, Rosenberg LE, eds. *Metabolic Control and Disease*. 8th ed. Philadelphia, PA: WB Saunders; 1980:1621–1693).

example, are all controlled from the CNS by the ANS. The sympathetic branch of the ANS is also structured to promptly address external threats to the integrity of the organism, by supporting the organism for "fight or flight," as described by Cannon early in the 20th century. Each preganglionic neuron of the SNS synapses with many postganglionic neurons in the sympathetic ganglia (average 1:20 pre to postganglionic cells), including neurons in ganglia above or below the level at which the preganglionic neuron exits the neuraxis. The adrenal medulla, furthermore, secretes E into the circulation thereby supporting the function of the SNS. That said, it is important to recognize that the SNS functions continuously

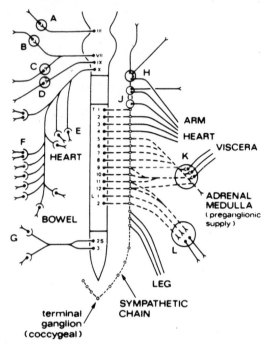

Parasympathetic system
from cranial nerves III, VII, IX, X
and from sacral nerves 2 and 3

Sympathetic system
from T1 to L2
preganglionic fibers ------
postganglionic fibers ———

A   ciliary ganglion
B   sphenopalatine (pterygopalatine)
    ganglion
C   submandibular ganglion
D   otic ganglion
E   vagal ganglion cells in heart wall
F   vagal ganglion cells in bowel wall
G   pelvic ganglia

H   superior cervical ganglion
J   middle cervical ganglion and
    inferior cervical (stellate) ganglion
    including T1 ganglion
K   coeliac and other abdominal
    ganglia
L   lower abdominal sympathetic
    ganglia

FIGURE 1.3. Organization of the peripheral autonomic nervous system. (From Moskowitz MS. Diseases of the autonomic nervous system. *Clin Endocrinol Metab.* 1977;6:745–768.)

in the regulation of normal physiology and that this regulation is characterized by discriminating rather than generalized responses.

Relationship between the sympathetic nervous system and the parasympathetic nervous system

The SNS and the parasympathetic nervous system (PSNS) are reciprocally related in terms of both activation and physiologic function. An increase in SNS

TABLE 1.5	Anatomic Organization of the Sympathetic and the Parasympathetic Nervous Systems
Sympathetic	**Parasympathetic**
Short preganglionic nerves	Long preganglionic nerves
Ganglia in paravertebral chains and preaortic area	Ganglia in innervated organs
Thoracolumbar outflow: preganglionic fibers originate in the intermediolateral cell column of the spinal cord, exit the spinal cord from T1–L2 and synapse in paravertebral and preaortic ganglia or the adrenal medulla	Craniosacral outflow: preganglionic fibers originate in the midbrain, the medulla oblongata exiting the neuraxis in cranial nerves III, VII, IX, X, and in the pelvic nerves from S2 to S4 regions of the spinal cord
Preganglionic dispersion: each preganglionic neuron synapses with many postganglionic sympathetic nerves	Much less preganglionic dispersion except for the vagal innervation of the enteric plexuses

TABLE 1.6	Chemical Neurotransmission in the Autonomic Nervous System: Adrenergic and Cholinergic Nerves	
	Sympathetic nervous system	**Parasympathetic nervous system**
Preganglionic nerves	Acetylcholine	Acetylcholine
Most postganglionic sympathetic nerves	Norepinephrine	Acetylcholine
Termination of action at neuroeffector junction	Reuptake into sympathetic nerve terminals	Hydrolysis by cholinesterase

activity is associated with a decrease in PSNS outflow and vice versa. The actions stimulated by SNS and the PSNS are also antagonistic. Pulse rate, for example, is increased by the SNS and decreased by the PSNS. Gut motility and secretion, similarly, are suppressed by the SNS and stimulated by the PSNS. This dual control of autonomic functions permits more precise regulation in the maintenance of homeostasis than would be possible with a unidirectional system.

Biosynthesis of Catecholamines

See Figure 1.6.

Biosynthetic pathway from L-tyrosine

Tyrosine is sequentially hydroxylated to 3,4-dihydroxyphenylalanine (DOPA), decarboxylated to DA, and hydroxylated at the β position to NE. The biosynthesis

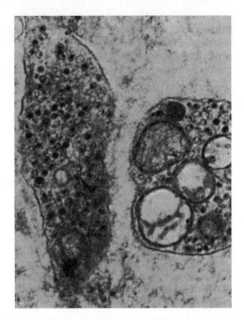

FIGURE 1.4. Electron photomicrograph of a sympathetic nerve ending in rat pineal gland. Note vesicles with electron-dense cores containing norepinephrine. Magnification ×45,000. (Courtesy of Dr. Floyd Bloom)

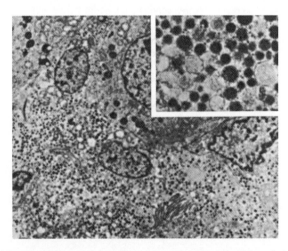

FIGURE 1.5. Electron photomicrograph of human adrenal medulla. Cells at the lower left containing small, electron-dense particles are adrenomedullary chromaffin cells with chromaffin granules; those above are adrenocortical cells. Magnification ×7,250. *Inset* shows chromaffin granules with clearly defined limiting membranes under higher magnification (×50,000). (Courtesy of Dr. James Connolly)

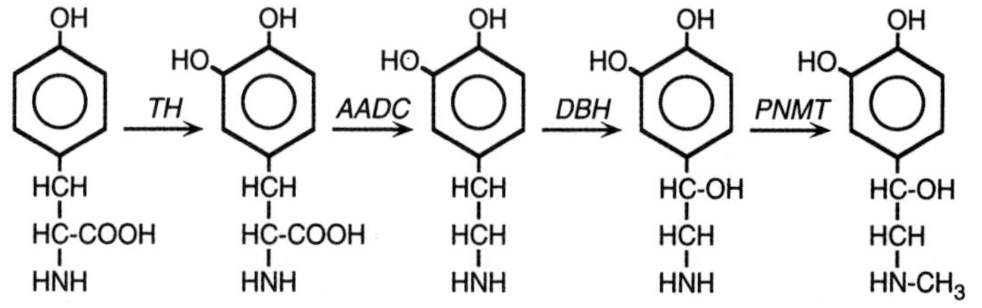

L-Tyrosine L-DOPA Dopamine L-Norepinephrine L-Epinephrine

FIGURE 1.6. Biosynthetic pathway for catecholamines. TH, AADC, and DBH catalyze formation of NE from tyrosine. Subsequent formation of E, catalyzed by PNMT, takes place in the adrenal medulla and in neurons of the CNS and peripheral ganglia that use epinephrine as a neurotransmitter. TH, tyrosine hydroxylase; AADC, aromatic-L-amino acid decarboxylase; DBH, dopamine β-hydroxylase; NE, norepinephrine; E, epinephrine; PNMT, phenylethanolamine-*N*-methyltransferase. (Modified from Levine RJ, Landsberg L. Catecholamines and the Adrenal Medulla. In: Bondy PK, Rosenberg LE, eds. *Duncan's Disease of Metabolism*. Philadelphia, PA: WB Saunders; 1974.)

of NE is carried out in peripheral adrenergic nerves and in central neurons that utilize NE as a neurotransmitter. In the chromaffin cells of the adrenal medulla, and certain neurons of the CNS, NE is *N*-methylated to E.

Catecholamine biosynthetic enzymes

Tyrosine hydroxylase (TH) is the rate-limiting step in catecholamine biosynthesis. The enzyme is localized to those peripheral tissues that synthesize and store catecholamines and those central neurons that utilize catecholamines as neurotransmitters. Tetrahydrobiopterin and Fe^{2+} are essential cofactors. The biosynthesis of NE and E is linked to release by changes in the activity of TH and, after prolonged stimulation, by the induction of TH synthesis. The coupling of synthesis and release assures a constant pool of stored NE or E despite wide variations in SA activity.

The DOPA formed by the action of TH on tyrosine is decarboxylated by **aromatic-L-amino acid decarboxylase (AADC)**, also known as DOPA decarboxylase, to form DA. Unlike the other enzymes involved in catecholamine biosynthesis AADC has a widespread distribution in non-neural tissues. The decarboxylation of circulating DOPA in the kidney to form DA, which then acts in autocrine or paracrine fashion to influence renal function, is an example of how a dopaminergic system might be involved in physiologic regulation.

In adrenergic neurons and the adrenal medulla, DA formed by the action of AADC in the cytoplasm is β-hydroxylated by **dopamine β-hydroxylase (DBH)** to form NE. This reaction, unique among the biosynthetic steps, occurs in the storage granules (dense core vesicles) of the SNS or chromaffin granules of the adrenal medulla. DBH, an enzyme that is similar to TH in many respects, uses ascorbate as a hydrogen donor; it is not substrate specific for DA, so it may hydroxylate a variety of phenylethylamines. The subcellular localization of DBH to the storage granules means that the final step in NE synthesis occurs within the storage site. DBH is both a structural component of the granule wall as well as a soluble component of the granule contents. The latter is released along with NE or E during SA activation, a fact accounting for the short-lived, and long gone, interest in plasma DBH as a marker of SA activity. Granular localization of DBH protects newly formed DA from degradation by cytoplasmic MAO.

In the adrenal medulla, NE is *N*-methylated to E by **phenylethanolamine N-methyltransferase (PNMT)**. S-adenosyl methionine is the methyl donor. In humans, about 80% of chromaffin cells synthesize and store E while the remainder store NE. The unique adrenal circulation that features a portal blood supply from the cortex to the medulla induces PNMT in the E-producing cells by exposing the chromaffin cells to very high levels of glucocorticoids. Interestingly, PNMT-positive chromaffin cells contain glucocorticoid receptors, while those lacking this enzyme do not. Although not required for differentiation of precursor cells into chromaffin cells, the capacity to produce E (at least in the adrenal medulla) does depend on the adjacent cortex and the steroid exposure that the portal system affords.

Note that PNMT is a cytosolic enzyme, so NE synthesized in the granules must diffuse out into the cytosol for conversion to E which is then taken up in the granule and stored. Although cumbersome, there is no feasible alternative to this sequence.

Another important point: although those chromaffin cells that produce E are phenotypically distinguishable from NE chromaffin cells, prolonged and intense adrenal medullary stimulation results in progressive decrease in E and increase in NE secretion, presumably due to a lack of time for regeneration of E stores in PNMT-positive cells. This means that in situations of strong adrenal medullary activation, the provenance of NE is uncertain; it cannot be assumed to derive from the SNS.

Regulation of catecholamine biosynthesis

In the sympathetic nerve endings and the adrenal medulla, the levels of NE and E respectively remain relatively constant despite wide variation in the degree of SA activity. This is accounted for in large measure by the coupling of catecholamine synthesis to catecholamine release, which is accomplished by increases in TH activity in the short term and by induction of TH synthesis in response to prolonged stimulation of SA activity. The increase in enzyme activity involves TH phosphorylation which alters the binding of catecholamines and tetrahydrobiopterin to the enzyme. The increase in enzyme biosynthesis with prolonged stimulation (termed "trans-synaptic induction") is related to increased Ach which reflects increased preganglionic impulse traffic. The importance of TH in maintaining NE stores in peripheral sympathetic nerve endings in the face of increased SNS activity is demonstrated by the depletion in tissue NE when TH is inhibited.

Catecholamine Storage and Release from Sympathetic Nerve Endings and Adrenal Medullary Chromaffin Cells

The sympathetic nerves

Sympathetic nerves originate from the paravertebral and preaortic ganglia (Fig. 1.3) (the latter are paravertebral ganglia that have migrated anterior to the aorta during embryonic development). These sympathetic ganglia receive a preganglionic innervation from cholinergic neurons in the intermediolateral cell column of the spinal cord (Fig. 1.2). The downward flow of impulse traffic from the CNS regulates catecholamine release from the sympathetic nerves which are small and unmyelinated; they are distributed to the vasculature and to viscera where the terminal sympathetic fibers innervate blood vessels, smooth muscle, and glands. Histochemical fluorescence studies of innervated tissues have demonstrated that the terminal sympathetic fibers form a syncytial network or ground plexus (Fig. 1.7) so that effector cells are innervated *en passant* with each nerve fiber serving many effector cells and each effector cell receiving innervation from several nerve fibers. Each terminal sympathetic fiber, furthermore, has numerous areas that form bulges or "varicosities" containing high concentrations of NE (Fig. 1.7).

Within the terminal sympathetic fibers, NE is stored in discrete subcellular vesicles that contain, by electron microscopy, a dense core. These dense core vesicles, or granules as they are sometimes called, contain approximately 15,000 molecules

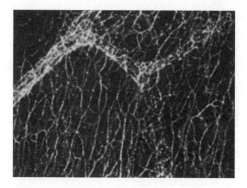

FIGURE 1.7.   Peripheral adrenergic nerve endings demonstrated by fluorescence histochemical technique. The ground plexus of terminal sympathetic fibers is shown in a normal rat iris. The plexus is particularly dense around a heavily innervated arteriole that courses through the field. Numerous discrete areas of high norepinephrine concentration (varicosities) are visible. Magnification ×160. (From Malmfors T. Studies on adrenergic nerves. *Acta Physiol Scand.* 1965;64(suppl 248):7–93.)

of NE. Each varicosity contains about 1,000 granules. Heavily innervated organs such as the heart have an NE concentration of about 1 µg per g of tissue. The concentration of NE in a given tissue is a measure of the density of sympathetic innervation. As noted above, NE concentration remains relatively constant despite different levels of sympathetic activity.

Sympathetic nervous system storage granules

Analogous to the chromaffin granules of the adrenal medulla, but considerably smaller and less complex, the dense core vesicles of the sympathetic nerve endings provide for the intracellular storage of the neurotransmitter NE (Fig. 1.4). In addition to NE, the granules contain the enzyme DBH, ATP, several neuropeptides, and a soluble protein involved in catecholamine storage called chromogranin A. The latter is one member of a family of proteins (chromogranins) that are useful as markers for neuroendocrine lineage. Uptake of amines into the granules is an active process requiring vesicular ATPase, resulting in an internal granule concentration of about 10,000 to 1 compared with the cytoplasm. The vesicular uptake process is not specific to catecholamines, a feature that in some circumstances may lead to the storage of "false neurotransmitters." Amines in the storage granules are protected from metabolism by MAO.

Chromaffin granules of the adrenal medulla

On average five to six times larger than the dense core vesicles of the sympathetic nerves, chromaffin granules contain soluble and membrane-bound DBH, ATP, chromogranin A, and neuropeptides (Fig. 1.8). The processes involved in catecholamine storage and release have been better studied in chromaffin granules than in sympathetic nerve endings and chromaffin granules; therefore, they have served as a model for the study of similar processes in the dense core vesicles of the SNS.

Release by exocytosis

Catecholamine release from both the adrenal medullary chromaffin cells and the sympathetic nerve endings is by exocytosis, a process by which the granule membrane fuses with the cell membrane and the entire soluble contents of the granule is extruded into the extracellular space (Fig. 1.9). Evidence for release by exocytosis includes the following: the soluble granule contents are released in proportion to their concentrations within the granule while cytoplasmic macromolecules are not released; the insoluble granule membranes are retained within the cell; and exocytotic figures have been demonstrated by electron microscopy. Depolarization of the chromaffin cell or the sympathetic nerve ending results in an influx of calcium which triggers the exocytotic process. In the case of the adrenal medullary chromaffin cell, Ach released from the splanchnic nerves results in depolarization; in the sympathetic nerve endings, the depolarization is caused by action potentials invading the terminal fibers. Docking regulatory proteins called SNAREs are involved in the fusion of granule and cell membrane at the initiation of the process.

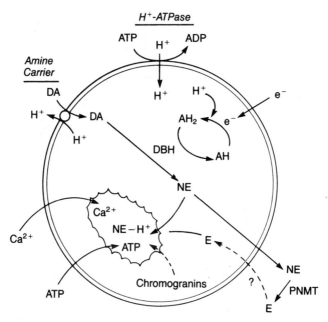

FIGURE 1.8.   Schematic representation of a chromaffin granule. The amine carrier for DA and other catecholamines, H$^+$-ATPase, electron shuttle (e$^-$) and uptake processes for calcium and ATP are shown in the granule membrane, along with a putative process for E uptake linked to NE egress. Stoichiometric relations are not shown. AH$_2$ refers to reduced ascorbate, which is an essential cofactor for DBH, which is regenerated by the electron shuttle. Calcium, ATP, catecholamines in protonated form, and chromogranins participate in a poorly understood storage complex. Synthesis of E occurs in the cytoplasm and therefore requires translocation of NE and uptake of E for storage within the granule. Although the energetics of a linkage between NE egress (down a huge concentration gradient) and E uptake appear to be quite favorable, conclusive evidence for such a process has not appeared. DA, dopamine; E, epinephrine; NE, norepinephrine; DBH, dopamine β-hydroxylase. (From Landsberg L, Young JB. Catecholamines and the Adrenal Medulla. In: *Williams Textbook of Endocrinology*, 9th ed. Philadelphia, PA: WB Saunders; 1998.)

Regulation of Central Sympathoadrenal Outflow

Although the basic wiring of the SA system permits generalized responses where these are required for the maintenance of homeostasis, it is abundantly clear that highly discriminating outflows to effector tissues continuously regulate basic autonomic functions such as pulse rate and blood pressure, cardiac output and blood flow distribution, respiration, energy production, and the like. These myriad functions are enabled by a constant flow of sensory information from peripheral tissues to the CNS; this information is carried in afferent nerve impulses and by changes in extracellular fluid substrate and hormone levels.

FIGURE 1.9. Schematic representation of catecholamine release from
a sympathetic nerve ending **(A)** and
from an adrenomedullary chromaffin
cell **(B)**. Catecholamines, DBH, ATP,
and chromogranin, as well as enkeph-
alins (not shown), are released in stoichiometric amounts from the storage
granule in response to nerve impulses.
E, epinephrine; NE, norepinephrine;
DBH, dopamine β-hydroxylase;
ACH, acetylcholine; ATP, adenosine
triphosphate. (From Landsberg L. The
sympathoadrenal system. In: Ingbar
SH, ed. *The Year in Endocrinology*.
New York, NY: Plenum 1976:291–344.)

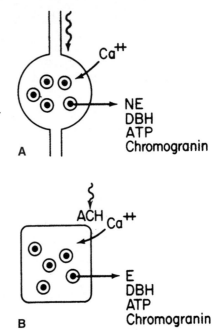

These signals are processed by specific regions of the brain where the responses
are integrated and changes in SA outflow generated in accordance with the needs
of the organism as a whole.

Afferent input to sympathoadrenal centers and efferent sympathoadrenal outflow

Neural afferents from the cranial nerves (particularly IX and X) and from the
spinal neurons at all levels of the neuraxis synapse in the nucleus of the solitary
tract (nucleus tractus solitarii, NTS) which projects the afferent information
both up and down the neuraxis where an integrated response is generated
(Tables 1.7 and 1.8).

The physical and chemical characteristics of the extracellular fluid are sampled
at the level of the hypothalamus which projects caudally to the brainstem sympathetic centers and directly to the preganglionic sympathetic neurons of the
spinal cord, and rostrally to forebrain structures including the cerebral cortex.
This sensing portion of the brain lies outside the blood brain barrier.

Efferent SA outflow is thus generated from the brainstem (particularly the
rostral ventral lateral medulla, RVLM) and from the hypothalamus. Integration
of responses occurs at many levels of the neuraxis including conscious centers
in the cortex, allowing for anticipation in the regulation of SA activity. As the

TABLE 1.7	Afferent Signals in the Regulation of SA Outflow
Neural afferents	
Integrated in the NTS	
Cranial nerves	
Arterial baroreceptors (pressure)	
Venous mechanoreceptors (volume)	
Spinal nerves	
Temperature	
Pain	
Extracellular fluid constituents	
Integrated in the hypothalamus	
Hormones	
Insulin	
Leptin	
Substrates	
Glucose	
Physical properties	
Temperature	
Osmolality	
Pao_2; $Paco_2$	

SA, sympathoadrenal; NTS, nucleus tractus solitarii; Pao_2, partial pressure of oxygen; $Paco_2$, partial pressure of carbon dioxide.

TABLE 1.8	Central SA Outflow
Brainstem sympathetic centers	
Tonically active neurons in the RVLM regulate CV system	
Receive afferents from the NTS, the hypothalamus, and the cerebral cortex	
Project to the spinal cord where they synapse with preganglionic sympathetic neurons in the intermediolateral cell column	
Hypothalamic SA centers	
Regulatory neurons receive afferent signals from the brainstem, the bloodstream, and the cerebral cortex	
Project to both the lower brainstem centers and directly to the preganglionic neurons in the spinal cord	

CV, cardiovascular, SA, sympathoadrenal; NTS, nucleus tractus solitarii; RVLM, rostral ventrolateral medulla.

brainstem SNS centers are tonically active, much of the regulation involves descending inhibition from rostral areas in the hypothalamus and elsewhere.

The Peripheral Dopaminergic System

In addition to its role as a precursor in the biosynthesis of NE and E, DA has a well-established role as a neurotransmitter in the CNS. It functions principally in the basal ganglia where it participates in the control of movement, and in the ventral tegmental area where it participates in the reward system of the brain and in the memory of poignant experiences via projections to the prefrontal cortex and the limbic system. Dopaminergic neurons originating in the arcuate and paraventricular nucleus of the hypothalamus project to the median eminence (the tuberoinfundibular pathway); DA released into the hypophyseal portal system tonically inhibits prolactin secretion from the anterior pituitary.

The fundamental structure of the DA system outside the CNS is more problematic. The situation may be summarized as follows: (1) DA receptors and a repertory of physiologic responses to DA are readily demonstrable particularly in the gut and kidneys. (2) DA is not a circulating hormone; levels in blood are below the threshold for stimulation of dopaminergic receptors. (3) There is scant evidence for dopaminergic nerves outside the CNS except for the special case of the carotid body where DA functions as an excitatory neurotransmitter for the type 1 glomus cells. And (4) DOPA, the immediate precursor of DA, circulates in plasma in high concentration and the DA-forming enzyme L-AADC has a widespread tissue distribution. The likely conclusion from these observations, therefore, is that DA is formed in peripheral tissues from the decarboxylation of circulating DOPA and that it acts as a paracrine or autocrine agonist in the effector tissues in which it is formed. The likely principal components of the peripheral dopaminergic system are therefore circulating DOPA and the enzyme L-AADC (Fig. 1.10).

Certain conceptual limitations of this formulation exist; for example, DA is formed intracellularly and yet it acts extracellularly since DA receptors are located on the cell membranes. This means that DA must escape metabolism by MAO and be transported out of the cell after synthesis to interact with DA receptors on the same (autocrine) or nearby (paracrine) cells. Nonetheless, there seems to be no alternative to this schema and the evidence that the system works like this in the kidney is reasonably strong. Two important questions about the dopaminergic system remain however: What is the origin of circulating DOPA

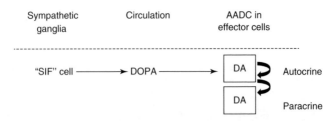

FIGURE 1.10. The peripheral dopaminergic system (hypothetical). See text for details. AADC, aromatic-L-amino acid decarboxylase; DOPA, 3,4-dihydroxyphenylalanine; DA, dopamine.

and how is the system regulated? Neither question can be answered definitively at the present time.

As TH has a limited distribution, it follows that DOPA must be synthesized in the neurally derived tissues that possess TH, thereby limiting the possibilities to the sympathetic nerve endings, the adrenal medullary chromaffin cells, the extra-adrenal chromaffin cells, and the small intensely fluorescent ("SIF") cells of the sympathetic ganglia. Origin from the SNS seems unlikely as chemical ablation of the SNS in animals is not accompanied by a fall in urinary DA leaving the extra-adrenal chromaffin cells and the SIF cells as possible sites of origin for circulating DOPA. How DOPA and the dopaminergic system are regulated remains a mystery. As DOPA levels are so high relative to DA levels, it seems unlikely that DOPA delivery can play a regulatory role and, similarly, the DOPA-forming enzyme L-AADC is widespread, present in excess, and not known to be regulated.

The small intensely fluorescent cells

It had been recognized since the late 19th century that sympathetic ganglia contained, in addition to the principal ganglion cells, groups of cells that resembled chromaffin cells rather than typical sympathetic neurons. It was subsequently demonstrated that these cells were intensely fluorescent when stained with formaldehyde, hence the name "small intensely fluorescent" cells. These cells are now known to contain granules that are bigger than those of typical sympathetic neurons but smaller than those of typical adrenal medullary chromaffin cells; DA is recognized to be the principal amine constituent of these SIF cells.

Although they continue to be mysterious, a fair amount has been learned about the SIF cells. In contrast to earlier opinions, the SIF cells are not precursors of the principal sympathetic ganglion cells; they follow a different developmental program (despite the fact that when exposed to nerve growth factor in vitro they develop neuronal markers). SIF cells, like the principal ganglion cells, receive a preganglionic innervation. Anatomic considerations suggest that SIF cells have features of both neurons and endocrine cells: some make synaptic connections with the ganglion cells as would be expected of an interneuron; others are nested near fenestrated capillaries suggesting endocrine access to the circulation at large. As DA is not a circulating hormone, it seems a reasonable hypothesis (as yet untested) that the SIF cell might be an important source of circulating DOPA. The preganglionic innervation of these cells would also provide a potential basis for physiologic regulation of a dopaminergic system by regulating DOPA influx into the circulation. This hypothetical schema is shown in Figure 1.10.

Metabolism and Termination of Action of Catecholamines

Catecholamines undergo enzymatic transformation to inactive metabolites, and are excreted in the urine. Locally released NE is actively taken up and restored to the sympathetic nerve endings (Fig. 1.11).

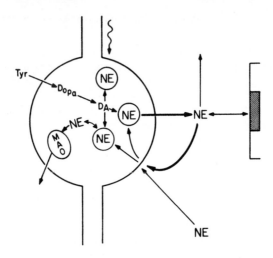

FIGURE 1.11.   Schematic representation of a sympathetic nerve ending. Tyr is taken up by the neuron and is sequentially converted to DOPA and DA; after uptake into the granule, DA is converted to NE. In response to nerve impulses, NE is released into the synaptic cleft, where it may diffuse into circulation or be recaptured by a nerve. Accumulation of extra-granular NE and DA is prevented by MAO. NE within the synaptic cleft also interacts with presynaptic (or prejunctional) α and β-adrenergic receptors on the axonal membrane that modulate NE release (not shown). A variety of other mediators also affect the presynaptic membrane and modulate NE release. Tyr, tyrosine; DOPA, 3,4-dihydroxyphenylalanine; DA, dopamine; NE, norepinephrine; MAO, monoamine oxidase. (From Landsberg L, Young JB. Catecholamines and the adrenal medulla. In: Bondy PK, Rosenberg LE, eds. *Metabolic Control and Disease*. 8th ed. Philadelphia, PA: WB Saunders; 1980;1621–1693.)

Metabolism by monoamine oxidase and catechol O-methyltransferase

Circulating NE and E are O-methylated to normetanephrine (NMN) and metanephrine (MN) respectively by catechol O-methyltransferase (COMT) in liver and kidney. MAO, widespread in tissues but particularly high in liver and kidney, deaminates the circulating MNs to 3-methoxy-4-dihydroxy-mandelic acid ("VMA") and the corresponding alcohol 3-methoxy-4-hydroxyphenylglycol (MHPG), both representing the final end products of NE and E metabolism.

MAO plays an important role in regulating the intraneural stores of NE by metabolizing cytosolic NE. Storage in the subcellular granules protects newly synthesized NE (as well as NE taken up from the synapses or circulation) from degradation.

The action of MAO and COMT on DA results in 3-methoxy-4-hydroxy phenylacetic acid (homovanillic acid, HVA).

The hydroxyl groups of the catechol molecule may also be conjugated in liver or gut with sulfate or glucuronide and excreted as conjugates. The designation

TABLE 1.9	**Excretion of Catecholamines and Metabolites in Urine Average 24-Hour Values and Sources**	
	Average daily excretion[a] **(µg/d)**	**Principal source(s)**
Epinephrine (E)	5	Adrenal medulla
Norepinephrine	30	Sympathetic nerve endings
Conjugated NE + E	100	Dietary catecholamines
Metanephrine (total)	65	Adrenal medulla
Normetanephrine (total)	100	Sympathetic nerve endings
3-methoxy-4-hydroxyman-elic acid (VMA)	4,000	SNS, adrenal medulla, CNS
3-methoxy-4-hydroxy-phenylglycol (MHPG)	2,000	SNS, adrenal medulla, CNS
Dopamine (DA)	225	Kidney
Homovanillic acid (HVA)	6,900	CNS

[a]Not upper limit.

"free" catecholamines in urine or plasma means unconjugated. The designation "total" means free + conjugated forms. Fractionated means separated into NE and E or NMN and MN. Catechols of dietary origin are conjugated in the gut and appear in urine as conjugates.

Daily average excretion of catecholamines and metabolites is shown in Table 1.9.

Inactivation by neuronal uptake

Neuronal uptake of catecholamines was discovered by Julius Axelrod and colleagues at the National Institutes of Health. These investigators, utilizing tritiated E and NE in laboratory rodents, demonstrated that after intravenous injection, catecholamines were rapidly cleared from the circulation but could be recovered unmetabolized from sympathetically innervated tissues hours later. These observations paved the way for recognition of neuronal uptake as the major mechanism of transmitter inactivation at adrenergic synapses; reuptake into the sympathetic nerve endings at neuroeffector junctions is the principal mechanism for termination of action of locally released NE (Fig. 1.11). The recaptured neurotransmitter enters the endogenous NE stores in the sympathetic nerve terminals.

The receptor for NE uptake on the neuronal axon has been cloned and demonstrated to possess 12 membrane-spanning domains. The uptake process is energy requiring and favors the naturally occurring L-isomer of catecholamines. It is distinct from the granule uptake mechanism of the sympathetic nerves and the adrenal medulla and is referred to as "uptake one" to distinguish it from the uptake of catecholamines ("uptake two") into non-neural cells. The neuronal uptake process is not specific to NE but is more avid for NE than E. Other sympathomimetic amines are also substrates for the neuronal uptake process.

The dynamics at the sympathetic nerve ending is shown in Figure 1.11. Locally released NE is (1) taken up by the nerve ending, (2) diffuses into the circulation, or (3) is metabolized in the effector tissue by COMT. NE that escapes reuptake enters the circulation where it constitutes the pool of plasma NE. Locally released NE that avoids reuptake and metabolism in the neuroeffector junction is commonly referred to as NE "spillover." Plasma NMN is derived from locally released NE metabolized to NMN in the effector tissue and from the metabolism of circulating NE by COMT in the liver. Uptake into the SN endings is the major mechanism of inactivation of locally released NE and the most important contributor to the clearance of circulating NE. Many commonly used drugs that affect autonomic nervous functions interact at the neuroeffector junction.

Adrenergic Receptors

Although it had been previously recognized by Sir Henry Dale that ergot alkaloids blocked the "excitatory" effects of E but not the inhibitory ones, and by Walter Cannon that the effects of sympathetic stimulation were both excitatory and inhibitory, it was Raymond Ahlquist in 1948 who first postulated the existence of two distinct adrenergic receptors which he designated α and β to correlate with the previously described inhibitory and excitatory effects. Ahlquist's postulation, based on the differential potency of a series of sympathomimetic amines on sympathetic responses, was strongly supported when specific antagonists of the β receptors (β blockers) were discovered. Subsequently, the field of adrenergic receptor biology has exploded with the elucidation of the molecular basis of receptor activation and the identification of major subtypes of both α and β receptors.

The structure of adrenergic receptors

Adrenergic receptors are cell surface proteins with an extracellular amino terminus, an intracellular carboxy terminus, and three membrane-spanning domains. The third intracellular loop and the carboxy terminus tail contain regulatory sites for phosphorylation that mediate changes in receptor action and underlie a part of "receptor desensitization" or tachyphylaxis.

Binding of the catecholamine to the adrenergic receptor initiates an intracellular cascade involving protein phosphorylation and ultimately resulting in characteristic tissue-specific responses. The second messenger for catecholamine receptors involves membrane-bound regulatory G proteins, so named because they bind guanosine triphosphate (GTP).

Adrenergic receptors coupled to G proteins

Binding of an adrenergic agonist to the adrenergic receptor stimulates the G proteins which in turn activate adenylyl cyclase or phospholipase C, membrane-associated enzymes that produce the intracellular second messengers cyclic AMP or inositol triphosphate (IP3) and diacylglycerol (DAG) (Fig. 1.12). The G protein associated with adenylyl cyclase may be stimulatory (Gs) or inhibitory (Gi), depending upon which receptor is occupied and leading to an increase or decrease in cyclic AMP, respectively (Fig. 1.12). The generation of cyclic AMP stimulates protein kinase A and other kinases. The stimulated kinases phosphorylate intracellular proteins that are the proximate cause of the cellular responses. The G protein associated with phospholipase C is designated Gq. The IP3 and DAG generated from activation of this enzyme increases intracellular calcium which acts as the second messenger by stimulating calcium/calmodulin protein kinases. An effect on intracellular calcium downstream from receptor activation, therefore, plays a critical role in coupling stimulation and response.

Alpha adrenergic receptors

NE and E have approximately equal potency as agonists of α_1 and α_2 receptors. Agonists and antagonists with specificity for the α_1 or α_2 receptor are available (Table 1.10). The classic physiologic response mediated by alpha receptors is

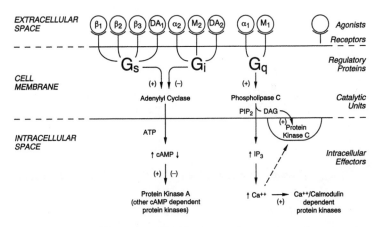

FIGURE 1.12.   Relations between autonomic agonists and receptors, membrane-bound regulatory proteins and enzymes, and intracellular effector systems. Adrenergic receptors are designated α and β, dopaminergic receptors DA, and muscarinic receptors M. Receptor subtypes are designated with subscripts 1, 2, and 3. "G" refers to the GTP-associated regulatory protein that stimulates (G$_s$) or inhibits (G$_i$) adenylate (adenylyl) cyclase or stimulates phospholipase C (Gq); (+), stimulation; (−), inhibition; PIP$_2$, phosphatidylinositol 4,5-biphosphate; DAG, diacylglycerol; IP$_3$, inositol 1,4,5-triphosphate. (Reproduced from Landsberg L, Young JB, Physiology and pharmacology of the autonomic nervous system. In: Wilson JD, Braunwald E, Isselbacher KJ, eds. *Harrison's Principles of Internal Medicine.* 12th ed. New York, NY: McGraw Hill, 1991:380–392, with permission of McGraw Hill.)

TABLE 1.10	α-**Adrenergic Receptors**	
	α_1	α_2
Agonist potency:	E = NE	E = NE
Selective agonist:	Phenylephrine	Clonidine
2nd messenger:	Gq → ↑ IP3, ↑ DAG, ↑ intracellular Ca^{2+}	Gi → ↓ cAMP ↑ or ↓ Ca^{2+} flux
Classic responses:	Vasoconstriction, intestinal relaxation, pupillary dilation	Prejunctional ↓ NE release, ↑ platelet aggregation, ↓ insulin secretion

E, epinephrine; NE, norepinephrine; IP3, inositol triphosphate; DAG, diacylglycerol; cAMP, cyclic adenosine monophosphate.

vascular smooth muscle contraction resulting in constriction of arterioles and veins. This effect on vascular smooth muscle is mediated by both α_1 and α_2 receptor subtypes, the α_1 response being the most important. Two receptors mediating vascular constriction provide the possibility of differential regulation as demonstrated in the subsequent section on thermoregulation. Other classic physiologic effects of α_1 receptors include intestinal relaxation, genitourinary sphincter contraction, and pupillary dilation.

α_2 receptors, in addition to vasoconstriction, classically mediate presynaptic inhibition of NE release from sympathetic nerve endings thus contributing to the dynamics at adrenergic synapses as described below. NE-induced platelet aggregation and SNS-mediated suppression of insulin release are other classic responses mediated by the α_2 receptor.

Beta adrenergic receptors

The classic physiologic effects mediated by the β receptor are cardiac stimulation, lipolysis, bronchodilation, and vasodilation (Table 1.11). β_1 receptor activation increases heart rate and force of cardiac contraction, lipolysis, and renin release

TABLE 1.11	β-**Adrenergic Receptors**		
	β1	β2	β3
Agonist potency:	NE = E	E >> NE	NE >> E
Selective agonist:	Dobutamine	Terbutaline	N/A
2nd messenger:	Gs → ↑ cAMP ↑ PKA	Gs → ↑ cAMP ↑ PKA	Gs → ↑ cAMP ↑ PKA
Classic responses:	↑ cardiac stimulation, ↑lipolysis, ↑ renin secretion	vasodilation, bronchodilation, ↑ glycogenolysis	↑ BAT heat production, ↑ lipolysis

NE, norepinephrine; E, epinephrine; cAMP, cyclic adenosine monophosphate; PKA, phosphokinase A; BAT, brown adipose tissue.

TABLE 1.12	**Dopaminergic Receptors**	
	DA1	DA2
Selective agonist:	Fenoldopam	Bromocriptine
2nd messenger:	Gs → ↑ cAMP ↑ PKA	Gi → ↓ cAMP ↓ PKA
Classic responses:	Vasodilation, ↑ Na excretion	↓ SNS ganglionic transmission, ↓ NE release (prejunctional), ↓ prolactin secretion

cAMP, cyclic adenosine monophosphate; SNS, sympathetic nervous system; NE, norepinephrine; PKA, phosphokinase A.

from the renal juxtaglomerular cells; β_2 receptor activation causes bronchodilation and vasodilation. The β_3 receptor regulates lipolysis in white adipose tissue and increases energy expenditure by stimulating lipolysis and heat production (mitochondrial respiration) in brown adipose tissue (BAT). E and NE are approximately equal in potency as agonists for the β_1 receptor whereas E is a much more potent agonist of the β_2 receptor. Specific pharmacologic agonists are available with selectivity for the β_1 and β_2 receptor, and an array of antagonists for the β_1 receptor and for both β_1 and β_2 (nonselective blockers) are available and in common clinical use. NE is a much more potent agonist for the β_3 receptor than E.

Physiologic responses to alpha and beta receptor activation

Many tissues are endowed with both alpha and beta receptors and in many cases the responses are antagonistic, for example arteriolar vasoconstriction and relaxation. In the physiologic situation which effect predominates? The balance between the numbers of each type of receptor in a particular tissue is of obvious importance, but in general, alpha receptor responses dominate at high agonist levels and beta responses at low agonist levels as beta receptor responses are more sensitive. Thus, very low doses of E cause vasodilation (beta mediated) whereas higher doses cause vasoconstriction (alpha mediated).

Dopaminergic receptors

The complex dopaminergic receptors (D-like) of the brain are related to the less complex DA receptors outside the CNS (Table 1.12). All dopaminergic receptors are coupled to G proteins (Fig. 1.12). In the periphery, DA1 receptors are located on non-neural tissues and mediate vasodilation in the renal, mesenteric, coronary, and cerebral vascular beds, as well as stimulating renal sodium excretion. DA2 receptors are located in autonomic ganglia, the SN endings, and the anterior pituitary where they inhibit ganglionic transmission, diminish NE release in response to impulse traffic (prejunctional modulation), and tonically inhibit prolactin secretion.

Alterations in adrenergic responsiveness: homologous and heterologous regulation

Sensitivity to the effect of any agonist may be defined as either the threshold concentration of agonist needed to produce a measurable response, and/or the concentration of agonist required to produce a half maximal response. Several factors alter the sensitivity of peripheral tissues to catecholamines; these depend upon changes induced in either the receptors themselves or in the downstream cascade of reactions leading to the physiologic response. The most important of these changes result in diminished responsiveness (loss of sensitivity) to the agonist, a phenomenon known as "desensitization" or "tachyphylaxis." The decrease in adrenergic effector cell responsiveness that occurs from adrenergic stimulation is referred to as "homologous" desensitization; this may be viewed as a mechanism to limit the intensity of prolonged stimulation on effector tissues and put a brake on adrenergic responses. The three processes underlying homologous desensitization include, in order of rapidity: (1) phosphorylation, which for cyclase-based receptors occurs on the third intracellular loop and the intracellular carboxy terminus of the receptor; (2) internalization or sequestration of the receptor which reduces receptor number; and (3) downregulation or deceased synthesis and increased destruction of the receptors which also reduce receptor number.

The underlying molecular mechanisms of homologous desensitization involving these three processes have been reasonably well characterized. A simplified version of these mechanisms of desensitization is as follows: (1) ligand (agonist) receptor occupancy couple receptor and cognate G protein stimulating second messenger kinases (Fig. 1.12); (2) the agonist stimulated receptor activates a G protein receptor kinase (GRK 2, previously identified as βARK) that relocates to the plasma membrane and phosphorylates serine and threonine residues on the receptor; (3) the phosphorylated G protein coupled receptor binds a cytoplasmic β-arrestin protein which markedly inhibits the signaling function of the G protein coupled receptor; (4) β-arrestin also initiates a series of reactions resulting in the internalization by endocytosis; (5) the internalized receptor is then either recycled to the cell membrane by phosphatases or destroyed by ubiquitination (downregulation). Allosteric modulators such as ions (Zn for example) and small peptides may also influence desensitization in positive or negative ways.

Of note, the β_3 receptor is unique in that it does not undergo desensitization in part because it lacks the long intracellular carboxy terminus with phosphorylation sites.

"Heterologous" regulation refers to changes in adrenergic responsiveness induced by factors other than adrenergic agonists. Examples include external temperature, pH, and the effects of hormones.

"Spare" receptors

As maximal responses to adrenergic agonists can be demonstrated at levels of receptor occupancy far below full occupancy, the question has arisen as to whether alterations in receptor number play a meaningful role in regulation of responsiveness. Because, by the law of mass reaction, the chances of interaction between agonist and receptor is greater when the receptor number is increased, it is logical to infer that the more "spare" receptors present the greater the sensitivity to a given amount of agonist. It has in fact been demonstrated that changes in receptor number are associated with alterations in sensitivity to the agonist.

Dynamics at the neuroeffector junction

The fate of NE released from the sympathetic nerve is recapture by the neuronal uptake process, metabolism by COMT in the effector tissue, and diffusion into the circulation where it constitutes the circulating pool of NE (Fig. 1.11). Reuptake into the nerve endings, quantitatively the most important, results in reintegration into the NE storage pool of the sympathetic nerve granules or less importantly, metabolism by neuronal MAO.

Prejunctional modulation of norepinephrine release

Although impulse traffic invading the terminal SN endings is the dominant force in determining how much NE is released, various other biologic ligands operating at the adrenergic neuroeffector junction have the potential to modulate NE release, the most physiologically relevant being catecholamines and Ach. Catecholamines via the α_2 receptor suppress NE release but via the β_2 receptor facilitate the release of NE. How to rationalize these two opposite effects is not entirely clear, but it is presumed that in the high synaptic NE concentration found in SN varicosities, the α-mediated suppression predominates. This may be yet another mechanism, in addition to homologous desensitization, to limit the intensity of SNS responses. It is also possible that circulating E, a much more potent agonist for the β_2 receptor than NE, might facilitate NE release under conditions of adrenal medullary stimulation.

Ach also exerts facilitatory prejunctional effects (nicotinic receptor) and suppressive effects (muscarinic receptor) on NE release with the inhibitory muscarinic effect predominating in vivo. In the heart, for example, vagal stimulation inhibits NE release. Cholinergic stimulation may also induce nitric oxide release which suppresses NE release.

Other factors affecting the prejunctional release of NE include adenosine which inhibits NE release. Adenosine in the adrenergic synapse may be derived from ATP released from SN endings along with NE during exocytosis.

Assessment of Sympathoadrenal Activity

Direct measurements of SA activity were not available until the 1980s when it became feasible to measure NE and E in plasma. Prior to that, measurements of catecholamines and metabolites in urine were used to diagnose pheochromocytoma but were not precise enough to reliably assess SA activity. As a consequence, the role played by the SA system in the regulation of normal physiologic processes and in the pathophysiology of a number of disease states could only be inferred from the effects produced by sympathetic blockade or by the application of adrenergic agonists. The availability of only these blunt instruments delayed the recognition of the role played by catecholamines in many circumstances; essential hypertension is an excellent example.

It is important to note that there is still no completely satisfactory way to assess the SA system. All currently available methods have limitations. Furthermore, assessment of SA activity is rarely useful in the clinic. Nonetheless, reliable assessment of SA activity remains critically important as a research tool. As potent, selective, and safe catecholamine agonists and antagonists are available for clinical use, understanding the role played by the SA system is central to full exploitation of their use in disease states and to the identification of useful therapeutic targets. This understanding can only be achieved by the assessment of SA activity in experimental studies involving humans and animal models.

The adrenal medulla

As the adrenal medulla is the only source of E (outside the CNS), assessment is relatively straightforward. Although plasma levels of E provide a measure of adrenal medullary activation, the usefulness of these levels is seriously compromised by the short plasma half-life, the sporadic nature of E secretion, and the technical limitations of detecting small changes within the normal range. Urinary E excretion gives a better integrated assessment over a 24-hour period or over discrete time periods in relation to physiologic perturbations. A research quality assay is required to detect small but meaningful changes within the range of normal.

The sympathetic nervous system: plasma levels of norepinephrine

Assessment of SNS activity is much more problematic for the following reasons: (1) NE is not a circulating hormone; it originates from sympathetic nerve endings throughout the body and constitutes that small fraction that escapes reuptake and metabolism. (2) SNS outflow is not homogeneous; increases in one organ system may not be accompanied by increases in others. (3) Under conditions of adrenal medullary stimulation, NE originates from the adrenal as well as the SNS. (4) As the levels of circulating NE are rapidly altered by changes in bodily position and anxiety, the acquisition of plasma samples for measurement of NE must be made under carefully controlled conditions; random levels by standard venipuncture are useless. The plasma half-life of NE is about 2 minutes.

Nevertheless, the above caveats to the contrary notwithstanding, measurements of plasma NE do provide useful information when obtained according to generally accepted protocols. The standard procedure entails 30 minutes of quiet rest in the supine position with the blood drawn through a previously placed i.v. line to avoid the perturbation of the venipuncture. Figure 1.13 demonstrates the provenance of the NE obtained from an indwelling catheter in an antecubital vein. As shown in the figure, the concentration of NE reflects the NE level in the arterial blood minus that extracted by SN endings in the forearm plus the NE added by the SN nerves downstream of the venipuncture. In general, venous NE levels

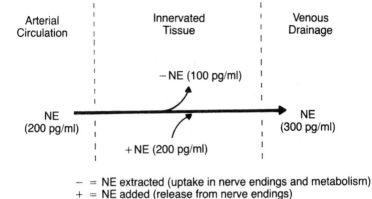

- = NE extracted (uptake in nerve endings and metabolism)
+ = NE added (release from nerve endings)

FIGURE 1.13. Relation between arterial and venous NE levels. The venous level depends on the amount of NE extracted as the innervated tissue is perfused with arterial blood and on the amount of NE released from nerve endings in response to neuronal impulse traffic in the area served by the venous drainage. Only a fraction of released NE escapes reuptake and local metabolism and diffuses into the venous circulation. Both the extraction process and diffusion from the region of the synapse are influenced by blood flow. To convert NE values to NMOL/L, multiply by 0.005911. NE, norepinephrine. (From Young JB, Landsberg L. Catecholamines. In: *Williams Textbook of Endocrinology*. 9th ed. Philadelphia, PA: WB Saunders; 1998.)

are about 30% higher than arterial levels and reflect importantly the addition of NE by the SNS in the area downstream of the catheter. The extraction of NE from the arterial blood perfusing the tissue is highly dependent on blood flow.

The plasma NE response to upright posture provides a convenient test of SNS function (Fig. 1.14). After 5 minutes of quiet standing the plasma NE concentration should double and a further increment should occur with isometric handgrip at about one-third maximal force. This test can also be performed on a tilt table. In patients with neurologic disorders affecting the SNS, the increment on standing or the basal level plus the increment are subnormal, as in idiopathic orthostatic hypotension. Note that this is the sole clinically useful test employing measurement of plasma NE.

Calculations of norepinephrine "spillover" rate

In an effort to improve the usefulness of plasma NE levels as indices of SNS activity in humans, infusions of tracer (tritiated) NE have been employed to calculate a rate of appearance of NE in the circulation. This is done by measuring the specific activity of NE in plasma under conditions of constant isotope infusion which corrects for changes in NE clearance that affect the measurement of plasma NE. Venous catheterization of different organs permits calculation of organ specific "spillover." As a research tool, studies utilizing these kinetic techniques have provided information incrementally better than assessments of plasma NE alone.

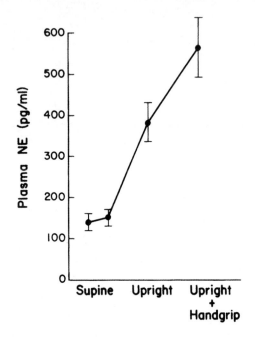

FIGURE 1.14.   Plasma NE responses to upright posture and isometric handgrip. Mean value ± SEM are shown for eight normal male subjects; supine values represent basal plasma NE levels. The increase in the plasma NE concentration after 5 min of quiet upright standing reflects activation of the SNS in response to orthostatic stress. A further increment in plasma NE is demonstrable after 5 min more of standing upright with isometric handgrip exercise at one-third maximal force. These maneuvers permit assessment of SNS reactivity. SNS, sympathetic nervous system; NE, norepinephrine. (From Landsberg L, Young JB. Sympathetic nervous system in hypertension. In: Brenner B, Stein JH, eds. *Hypertension: Contemporary Issues in Nephrology*. Vol. 8. New York, NY: Churchill Livingstone; 1981:100–141.)

Urinary norepinephrine excretion

Twenty-four–hour NE excretion provides a useful measure of integrated SNS activity, and with research, quality assays have provided useful information in both clinical and population-based studies. The amount of NE excreted in the urine is equal to the amount filtered at the glomerulus minus the amount metabolized and extracted by the renal parenchyma plus the amount added by the renal sympathetic nerves.

Microneurography

Transcutaneous placement of electrodes in sympathetic nerves with recording of impulse frequency and amplitude provides a direct means of determining sympathetic outflow to skeletal muscle blood vessels in unanesthetized humans with the output described as muscle sympathetic nerve activity. Recordings are usually made from the peroneal nerve. Significant limitations of this technique include the fact that it is invasive and technically demanding and that it measures SNS activity over a relatively short time period. Much useful information, however, has been developed by the skillful application of nerve recordings and the results have clarified the role of the SNS in the pathogenesis of a variety of disease states. The technique is also applicable to the study of the SNS in anesthetized animals.

Norepinephrine turnover rate in the tissues of laboratory rodents

Tracer doses of tritiated 3HL-NE, when administered i.v. to unanesthetized rats, is taken up by SN endings throughout the body where it equilibrates the endogenous NE stores, and is released along with endogenous NE in response to SN impulse traffic (Fig. 1.15). Once the NE stores are labeled with tracer, the animals are returned to their cages and groups are killed at preselected times over a 24-hour period and the tissues of interest harvested and analyzed for tritiated and endogenous NE. As shown in Figure 1.16 the decline in specific activity of NE (reflecting neurotransmitter release) follows first-order kinetics. This monoexponential decline permits calculation of a slope which represents the fractional turnover rate of NE and the product of the fractional turnover rate, and the endogenous NE concentration represents the actual amount of NE released per gram of tissue per hour over the time period as shown in Figure 1.16.

This technique permits comparison of SNS activity in various physiologic or pathophysiologic conditions as shown in Figure 1.17, which demonstrates the effect of 24 hours of cold exposure on SNS activity in heart. The increased SNS activation is shown graphically by the line of steeper slope. This technique also permits demonstration of suppressed SNS activity, difficult to show by other techniques, and allows assessment of the SNS independent of activity of the

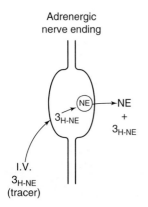

FIGURE 1.15. Labeling NE stores in SN endings. NE, norepinephrine. (From Landsberg L. *Cell Mol Neurobiol.* 2006;26(4–6):497–508.)

Adrenergic
nerve ending

NE
+
3_{H-NE}

3_{H-NE}

I.V.
3_{H-NE}
(tracer)

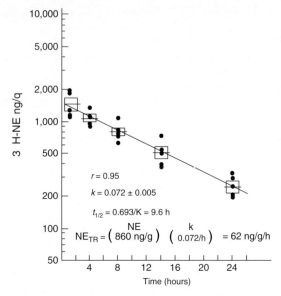

FIGURE 1.16.   Determination of NE turnover rate. NE, norepinephrine. (From Landsberg L. *Cell Mol Neurobiol.* 2006;26(4–6):497–508.)

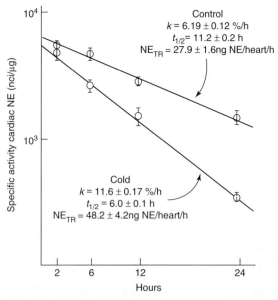

FIGURE 1.17.   Effect of cold on cardiac NE turnover. NE, norepinephrine. (From Landsberg L. *Cell Mol Neurobiol.* 2006; 26(4–6):497–508.)

adrenal medulla. Arduous and technically demanding, this technique has proved extraordinarily useful in studying the SNS.

BIBLIOGRAPHY BY CATEGORY

HISTORY

Bennett MR. One hundred years of adrenaline: the discovery of autoreceptor. *Clin Auton Res*. 1999;9:145–159.

GENERAL

Westfall TC, Westfall DP. Neurotransmission: The Autonomic and Somatic Motor Nervous Systems. In: Brunton LL, Chabner BA, Knollmann BC, eds. *Goodman & Gilman's The Pharmacological Basis of Therapeutics*. New York, NY: McGraw Hill; 2011.

DEVELOPMENT

Huber K. The sympathoadrenal cell lineage: specification, diversification, and new perspectives. *Dev Biol*. 2006;298:335–343.

Huber K, Kalcheim C, Unsicker K. The development of the chromaffin cell lineage from the neural crest. *Auton Neurosc: Basic Clin*. 2009;151:10–16.

CHROMAFFIN CELLS

Unsicker K, Krieglstein K. Growth factors in chromaffin cells. *Prog Neurobiol*. 1996;48:307–324.

STORAGE AND RELEASE

Jahn R. Principles of exocytosis and membrane fusion. *Ann NY Acad Sci*. 2004;1014:170–178.

Winkler H. The adrenal chromaffin granule: a model for large dense core vesicles of endocrine and nervous tissue. *J Anat*. 1993;183:237–252.

DOPAMINE—SIF CELLS

Eränkö O. Small intensely fluorescent (SIF) cells and nervous transmission in sympathetic ganglia. *Ann Rev Pharmacol Toxicol*. 1978;18:417–410.

Hall AK, Landis SC. Principal neurons and small intensely fluorescent (SIF) cells in the rat superior cervical ganglion have distinct developmental histories. *J Neurosci*. 1991;11:472–484.

Iturriaga R, Alcayaga J, Gonzalez C. Neurotransmitters in carotid body function: the case of dopamine [Invited Article]. Arterial Chemoreceptors, of the Series. *Adv Exp Med Biol*. 2009;648:137–143.

Matthews MR. Small, intensely fluorescent cells and the paraneuron concept. *J Electron Microsc Technol*. 1989;12:408–416.

Peterson SM, Urs N, Caron MG. Dopamine receptors (Chapter 13). In: Roberston D, Biaggioni I, Burnstock G, et al., eds. *Primer on the Autonomic Nervous System*. New York, NY: Elsevier;2012.

REGULATION of SYMPATHOADRENAL

Benarroch EE. Central autonomic control (Chapter 2). In: Roberston D, Biaggioni I, Burnstock G, et al., eds. *Primer on the Autonomic Nervous System*. New York, NY: Elsevier; 2012:9–12.

Morrison SF. Differential control of sympathetic outflow. *Am J Physiol Regul Integr Comp Physiol* 2001;281:R683–R698.

Souvatzoglou A. The sympathoadrenal system: integrative regulation of the cortical and the medullary adrenal functions (Chapter 4). In: Linos D, van Heerden JA, eds. *Adrenal Glands*. Berlin, Germany: Springer; 2009:33–39.

Young JB, Landsberg L. Synthesis, storage, and secretion of adrenal medullary hormones: physiology and pathophysiology (Chapter 1). In: *Handbook of Physiology, The Endocrine System, Coping with the Environment: Neural and Endocrine Mechanisms*. London: Wiley; 2001.

G-PROTEINS

Gilman AG. G proteins: transducers of receptor-generated signals. *Ann Rev Biochem*. 1987;56:615–649.

Lodish H, Berk A, Zipursky SL, et al. G protein-coupled receptors and their effectors. In: *Molecular Cell Biology*. 4th ed. New York, NY: W.H. Freeman; 2000.

RECEPTOR REGULATION

Freedman NJ, Liggett SB, Drachman DE, et al. Phosphorylation and desensitization of the human β_1-adrenergic receptor. *J Biol Chem*. 1995;270:17953–17961.

Khoury E, Clément S, Laporte SA. Allosteric and biased G protein-coupled receptor signaling regulation: potentials for new therapeutics. *Front Endocrinol*. 2014.doi:10.3389/fendo.2014.00068.

Kohout TA, Lefkowitz RJ. Regulation of G protein-coupled receptor kinases and arrestins during receptor desensitization. *Mol Pharmacol*. 2003;63:9–18.

Krasel C, Bünemann M, Lorenz K, et al. β-Arrestin binding to the β_2-adrenergic receptor requires both receptor phosphorylation and receptor activation. *J Biol Chem*. 2005;280:9528–9535.

Lefkowitz RJ. G protein-coupled receptors. *J Biol Chem*. 1998;273:18677–18680.

Luttrell LM, Lefkowitz RJ. The role of β-arrestins in the termination and transduction of G-protein-coupled receptor signals. *J Cell Sci*. 2002;115:455–465.

Tobin AB. G-protein-coupled receptor phosphorylation: where, when and by whom. *Br J Pharmacol*. 2008;153(suppl 1):S167–S176.

Yanamala N, Klein-Seetharaman J. Allosteric modulation of G protein coupled receptors by cytoplasmic, transmembrane and extracellular ligands. *Pharmaceuticals*. 2010;3:3324–3342.

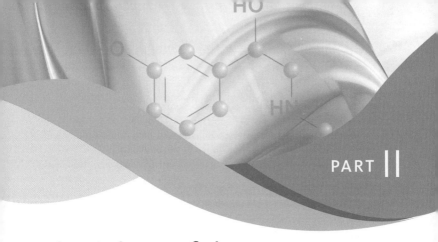

PART II

Physiology of the
Sympathoadrenal System

General and Unique Features of Regulation by the Sympathoadrenal System: Central Neural Control

The autonomic nervous system is the means by which the brain regulates physiologic processes in accord with the needs of the organism as a whole. In concert, the sympathetic and the parasympathetic nervous systems regulate cardiovascular, metabolic, and visceral functions to maintain homeostasis and provide the means for dealing with acute and chronic changes in the external environment.

Integrated responses

The hypothalamus receives neural afferents from blood vessels and viscera and samples the blood for hormones, substrates, ions, tonicity, and the like. SA outflow is adjusted to maintain the adequacy of the circulation, the provision of substrates for metabolizing tissues, and the appropriate level of visceral function. An example of hypothalamic integration may be illustrated in the response elicited by volume depletion. A fall in venous return triggers an increase in SNS outflow to the venous capacitance vessels, with the resultant venoconstriction increasing central blood volume. If the decrease in venous return is sufficiently great to cause a fall in blood pressure, the arterial baroreceptors trigger an increase in outflow to the resistance portion of the circulation, resulting in arteriolar vasoconstriction. At the same time, an increase in renin secretion is stimulated by the SNS, resulting in enhanced aldosterone secretion and the consequent increase in renal sodium reabsorption. Also at the level of the hypothalamus, the decrease in venous return changes the relationship between vasopressin release and plasma tonicity so that more vasopressin is secreted at lower tonicity of the body fluids. The vasopressin response maintains the circulating plasma volume (albeit at a lower serum sodium) and supports arteriolar vasoconstriction. Thus, the integration within the hypothalamus results in coordinated changes in SNS outflow along with appropriate endocrine adaptation that supports the circulation. These changes reflect the redundancy and the hierarchy that characterize sympathetic responses.

Generalized versus discriminant responses

Generalized SA discharge is most dramatic in the classic "fight or flight" response. These striking cardiovascular and metabolic changes first described by Walter Cannon permit rapid adaptation to abrupt environmental challenges. This should not, however, obscure the fact that the SA system is tonically active regulating blood flow distribution, cardiac output, substrate supply, and energy expenditure, to highlight but a few of the many functions that reflect the continuous discriminating outflow from the SA system.

Speed and anticipation

As an efferent limb of the CNS, sympathetic responses are rapid in comparison with the slower effects induced by circulating hormones. Connections between the integrative centers in the hypothalamus, the tonically active brainstem centers, and the cerebral cortex provide the anatomic and neurophysiologic basis for conscious influence on autonomic functions. Among other things, these connections enable anticipation a role in physiologic regulation. It has been shown, for example, that in runners competing in a race, plasma renin rises before the race actually begins. This change, mediated by the SNS, defends against volume depletion in anticipation of strenuous exertion, thereby lessening the impact of the upcoming activity on the circulation and protecting the integrity of the internal environment.

Relationship between the sympathetic nervous system and adrenal medulla

It is well established, although not sufficiently appreciated, that the adrenal medulla and the SNS are regulated independently. Although these two limbs of the SA system always function in a coordinated manner, the activation is not always congruent. The classic view, best enunciated by Walter Cannon, is that the adrenal medulla supports the functions of the SNS with circulating E under conditions of "fight or flight." Activation of both the adrenal medulla and the SNS is noted with exertion and cold exposure. There are, however, many situations in which the SNS is suppressed and the adrenal medulla is stimulated, such as hypoglycemia and severe trauma. The physiologic significance of this dissociation is discussed in subsequent sections.

Direct and indirect effects

In addition to the direct effect exerted by catecholamines on adrenergic receptors, several indirect effects also contribute to the physiologic responses regulated by the SA system. These indirect effects include changes in blood flow, catecholamine-mediated changes in the secretion of other hormones, and the provision of substrate for metabolizing tissues. For example, during physical exercise, SA stimulation not only increases cardiac output directly but also distributes blood flow to the musculature; mobilizes substrates by stimulating glycogenolysis and lipolysis; suppresses insulin that aids in substrate mobilization; and stimulates renin that helps maintain plasma volume. The indirect effects reinforce the direct ones.

Cardiovascular Effects of the Sympathoadrenal System

SA control of the circulation regulates the cardiac output, oversees the distribution of blood flow, and maintains the perfusion pressure of critical organs. It achieves this by regulating cardiac contractility and heart rate, and venous and arteriolar vasoconstriction (Table 2.1; Fig. 2.1).

Afferent neural pathways

Well-developed mechanisms, in the form of mechanoreceptors, assess changes in pressure and relay these changes to the nucleus of the solitary tract (NTS) via the IXth and Xth cranial nerves. There are, however, no mechanisms that permit direct assessment of plasma volume. A surrogate, therefore, is utilized to determine volume status, namely changes in pressure in the capacitance (low-pressure) portion of the circulation. Mechanoreceptors in the great veins, pulmonary veins, and right atrium transmit impulses in cranial nerve X; an increase in pressure stimulates an increase in impulse traffic, which registers as adequate filling pressure and diminishes SNS outflow to the veins; a decrease in pressure indicates a fall in venous return and initiates an increase in SNS-mediated venoconstriction, which returns blood from the low-pressure portion of the circulation to the central pool, thereby restoring venous return.

TABLE 2.1 **Cardiovascular Effects of the SA System**
Cardiac effects (β_1 mediated)   ↑ contractility   ↑ rate   ↑cardiac output   ↑ myocardial oxygen consumption
Vascular effects (α_1 and α_2 mediated)   ↑ arterial, arteriolar, and venoconstriction
Effects on renin release (β_1 mediated)   ↑ A II, aldosterone
Net effects   ↑ cardiac output   ↑ blood pressure

SA, sympathoadrenal; A II, angiotensin II.

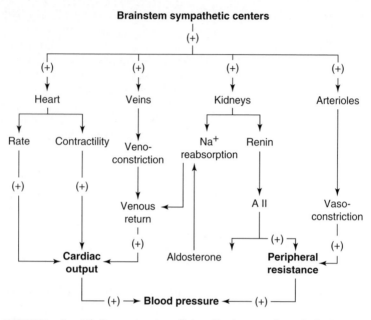

FIGURE 2.1.   Sympathetic nervous system effects on blood pressure. Sympathetic stimulation (+) increases blood pressure by effects on the heart, the veins, the kidneys, and the arterioles. The net result of sympathetic stimulation is an increase in both cardiac output and peripheral resistance. A II, angiotensin II (From Young JB, Landbserg L. Obesity and Circulation. In: Sleight P, Jones JV, eds. Scientific Foundations of Cardiology. London, Heinemann, 1983.)

The arterial baroreceptors, located principally in the aorta and carotid arteries, respond directly to changes in arterial pressure; mechanoreceptors in the adventitia of the arteries transmit impulses via the IXth and Xth cranial nerves to the NTS. Increases in BP suppress SNS outflow, whereas decreases stimulate SNS, resulting in arteriolar vasoconstriction and increased heart rate.

The response to upright posture

With standing, the fall in venous return decreases impulse traffic from the receptors in the great veins; at the level of the NTS, this decrease releases the tonic inhibition on the lower SNS centers, thereby increasing SNS outflow, causing venoconstriction that maintains venous return and prevents a fall in BP. If the arterial pressure dips, the arterial (high-pressure) mechanoreceptors come into play. Decreased impulse traffic, transmitted to the NTS, disinhibits the lower brainstem centers, resulting in enhanced SNS outflow, consequent arteriolar vasoconstriction, and an increase in heart rate. The smooth functioning of this system, operating continuously, prevents significant postural changes in blood pressure. The changes in SNS outflow are, of course, more pronounced in exigent situations such as severe volume depletion or hemorrhage.

Regulation by descending inhibition

The operation of this system demonstrates an important additional feature of SNS regulation: control by descending inhibition. Tonically active lower centers are under constant restraint from above, and regulation is achieved by modulating that restraint. This is an important principle of SNS regulation, presaged by the experiments of Sir Charles Sherrington in the late 19th century.

Additional afferent signals regulating sympathetic nervous system outflow to the circulation

Changes in the partial pressure of oxygen, carbon dioxide, pH, insulin, glucose, leptin, angiotensin II, among others, all affect SNS outflow from the brainstem (RVLM) to the circulatory system. These are described in the appropriate sections that follow.

Direct circulatory effects of sympathetic nervous system stimulation

The predominant direct effect of catecholamines on the heart is postjunctional β_1-mediated cardiac stimulation (Fig. 2.1). Heart rate is increased (+ chronotropic effect), as is contractility (+ inotropic effect) and conduction velocity. The net effect is to increase cardiac output at the expense of increased myocardial oxygen consumption, which depends importantly on rate and contractile state (Table 2.1).

Vasoconstriction involving arteries and veins is the major effect of catecholamines on the vasculature. Both the α_1 and α_2 receptors mediate vascular smooth muscle contraction, but significant heterogeneity in the disposition of receptor subtypes exists depending on the vascular bed, size of artery, and location of veins. Large arteries, in general, possess α_1 receptors, deep veins favor α_1 receptors, and both receptor subtypes mediate constriction in the arteriolar resistance vessels. There appears to be a regulatory component to the disposition of α receptor subtypes in veins: α_1 receptors predominate in deep veins, and these are associated with diminished responsiveness to NE in the cold; α_2 receptors are more prevalent in the superficial veins, and cold enhances α_2 responses in the superficial venous system. The net result of these changes is shunting of blood to the deep system during cold exposure, thus conserving heat, rather than dissipating it to the environment.

Indirect circulatory effects of the sympathetic nervous system

SNS stimulation enhances venous return by venoconstriction, by a direct effect to enhance renal tubular sodium reabsorption, and by stimulation of renin release with the generation of angiotensin II and an increase in aldosterone.

The sympathoadrenal system is not associated with significant vasodilation

Although controversy has existed about the role, if any, of sympathetically mediated vasodilation, it is clear that in humans that role is inconsequential at best. Evidence for cholinergic vasodilatory neurons within the sympathetic outflow in humans is scant to nonexistent. β_2-mediated vasodilation is demonstrable in the presence of α blockade, but in unblocked subjects it occurs only at very low circulating levels of E. The local release of nitrous oxide in stimulated tissues may account for some of the vasodilatory effects attributed to catecholamines.

Taken together, the effects of catecholamines on the cardiovascular system increase cardiac output, increase blood pressure, and increase myocardial oxygen consumption (Table 2.1).

Metabolic Effects of the Sympathoadrenal System

The effects of catecholamines on metabolism are manifold and include, most importantly, substrate mobilization and heat production. The former involves the breakdown of stored nutrients in the form of glycogen and triglycerides into utilizable substrates (glucose, lactose, free fatty acids) and the latter the uncoupling of respiration in BAT mitochondria so that heat generation results rather than ATP synthesis.

The important fuel depots for stored nutrients include liver, adipose tissue, and skeletal muscle (Table 2.2). In general, the substrate-mobilizing processes regulated by the SA system depend on the balance between catecholamines and insulin (Fig. 2.2), and reflect both direct and indirect effects.

Sympathoadrenal effects on hepatic glucose output

A prime function of the liver is to maintain circulating glucose levels during fasting and to provide extra glucose in situations of urgent need ("fight or flight"). This is accomplished by glycogenolysis in the presence of sufficient glycogen stores and by gluconeogenesis when hepatic glycogen is depleted. The β_2 receptor operating through cyclic adenosine monophosphate (cAMP) activates the hepatic phosphorylase that cleaves glucose moieties from glycogen. This appears to be the major mechanism in humans, although an α_1 receptor non-cAMP process is also associated with glycogenolysis. Circulating E is the principal catecholamine

TABLE 2.2	Substrate Mobilization by Catecholamines
Liver	
↑ hepatic glucose output (predominantly β_2 receptor)	
glycogenolysis → glucose from glycogen breakdown	
gluconeogenesis → glucose synthesized from lactate, alanine, glutamine, glycerol	
Adipose tissue	
↑ lipolysis → free fatty acids, glycerol (predominantly β_1, β_3 receptor)	
Skeletal muscle	
↑ glycogenolysis→ lactate (β_2 receptor)	

Predominantly circulating E rather than the SNS; insulin exerts opposing effects; net result on substrate mobilization is a balance between E and insulin and is highly dependent on the physiologic situation.
SNS, sympathetic nervous system; E, epinephrine.

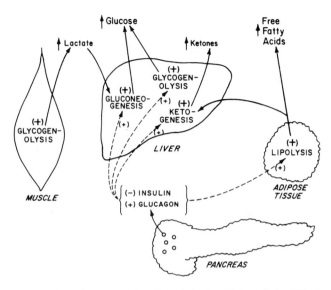

FIGURE 2.2.   Schematic representation of catecholamine effects on fuel mobilization in liver, adipose tissue, and skeletal muscle. Direct effects are reinforced by (but do not require) catecholamine-mediated suppression of insulin and stimulation of glucagon. (+), stimulation; (-), inhibition. (From Landsberg L, Young JB. Catecholamines and the adrenal medulla. In: Bondy PK, Rosenberg LE, eds. *Metabolic Control and Disease.* 8th ed. Philadelphia: WB Saunders, 1980:1621–1693.)

stimulating glycogenolysis; glucagon also enhances glycogenolysis, whereas insulin inhibits glycogenolysis and promotes glycogen synthesis.

The hepatic glycogen store, about 100 g, is largely depleted by glycogenolysis occurring during an overnight fast; under these circumstances, hepatic glucose output is maintained by gluconeogenesis. Both E and glucagon increase hepatic gluconeogenesis via a cAMP mechanism; insulin antagonizes gluconeogenesis by accelerating the breakdown of cAMP via phosphodiesterase.

Sympathoadrenal effects on lipolysis in white adipose tissue

Adipose tissue is the major energy repository in humans, comprising approximately 10 to 15 kg in healthy nonobese adults. As is the case with hepatic glucose output, catecholamines and insulin are the major regulators of lipolysis in white adipose tissue, playing opposing roles in stimulating and suppressing the release of free fatty acids. SA regulation of lipolysis is principally by E, but the SNS may also be involved in some situations.

Stimulation of lipolysis in white adipose tissue is a defining action of the β_1 adrenergic receptor. The β_3 adrenergic receptor, the mediator of lipolysis in BAT, is also expressed on white fat cells and stimulates lipolysis in white fat as well as BAT.

Catecholamines stimulate lipolysis by activating hormone-sensitive lipase, an action that depends upon adenylyl cyclase and cAMP-dependent protein kinase A. Phosphorylation of hormone-sensitive lipase activates the enzyme; dephosphorylation, stimulated by insulin, inactivates it, thereby exerting an antilipolytic effect.

The products of lipolysis, free fatty acids and glycerol, are processed in the liver to lipoproteins, when insulin levels are high, and to ketone bodies, when insulin is low or absent. Ketogenesis is highly dependent on the flow of free fatty acids to the liver, so catecholamine-induced lipolysis plays a major role in ketone formation. The glycerol liberated from adipose tissue is also a substrate for both triglyceride formation and gluconeogenesis in the liver.

Sympathoadrenal effects on glycogenolysis in skeletal muscle

Although the glycogen concentration in liver is much higher than in skeletal muscle, the total glycogen stored in muscle is greater because of the large muscle mass. Glycogenolysis in muscle, stimulated by the β_2 adrenergic receptor in response to circulating E, provides a rapidly available source of glucose for exercising muscle. Because muscle lacks the enzyme glucose-6-phosphatase, breakdown of glycogen in muscle does not supply glucose to the circulation. Glucose-6-phosphate is metabolized in muscle to pyruvate and lactate; lactate released into the circulation may be converted in the liver to glucose (gluconeogenesis), which enters the circulation and may be returned to muscle in what is known as the "Cori cycle."

Sympathetic Nervous System Effects on Heat Conservation and Heat Generation

The role of the SNS in mammalian thermoregulation includes both a cardiovascular and metabolic component. These effects are described fully in sections that follow on thermoregulation and cold exposure. The basic mechanisms involve heat conservation or heat dissipation by changes in blood flow to the extremities and the generation of metabolic heat by the stimulation of BAT.

Heat conservation and dissipation

α_1- and α_2-mediated vasoconstriction diminishes blood flow to the extremities and shifts venous return from the superficial veins of the limbs to the deep venous system, which forms a plexus around the arteries, thereby returning heat from the arterial blood to the central pool. This deep venous system forms a countercurrent system for efficient heat transfer. The opposite changes, vasodilation, from withdrawal of sympathetic tone effectively dissipate heat to the environment.

Heat production in brown adipose tissue

A highly specialized tissue for the generation of heat, BAT has long been recognized as a thermogenic organ in small mammals such as laboratory rodents and

TABLE 2.3	**Brown and White Adipose Tissue**
Brown adipose tissue	**White adipose tissue**
Function: heat production	Function: fuel (triglyceride) storage
Mitochondria: densely packed	Mitochondria: sparse
Sympathetic innervation: dense	Sympathetic innervation: sparse
Lipolysis: β_3 mediated	Lipolysis: β_1 and β_3 mediated
NE: principal physiologic ligand	E: principal physiologic ligand
Respiration uncoupled (UCP 1)	Respiration normally coupled (no UCP 1)

NE, norepinephrine; E, epinephrine; UCP, 1uncoupling protein.

in human neonates; only recently, however, has a potentially significant role for BAT in adult humans been generally acknowledged. A resurgence of interest in BAT was triggered by PET scans obtained from patients undergoing evaluation of malignancies. Isotope uptake around the neck and upper mediastinum in some of the patients was shown to be BAT by both histologic and biochemical techniques.

Some of the differences between white adipose tissues and BATs are summarized in Table 2.3.

The regulation of BAT heat production has been extensively studied, and the underlying mechanisms are reasonably well understood (Fig. 2.3). The SNS, via the β_3 adrenergic receptor, activates heat production by initiating a cascade

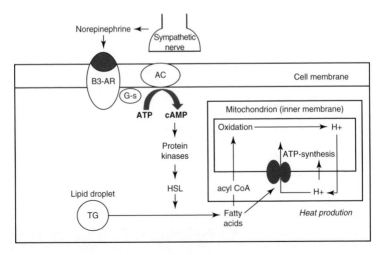

FIGURE 2.3. BAT stimulation. See text for details.

that begins with adenylyl cyclase and cAMP stimulation of lipolysis. The free fatty acids liberated by the activation of hormone-sensitive lipase in BAT serve as substrates for oxidation in BAT mitochondria and as activators of uncoupling protein (UCP 1). Also known as "thermogenin," UCP 1 is a mitochondrial carrier protein that is activated by free fatty acids and that plays a critical role in uncoupling BAT mitochondria. Uncoupling means that substrate oxidation, exothermic reactions that release the energy stored in nutrients, proceeds without ATP synthesis. In the normally coupled state, substrate oxidation is tightly coupled to ATP synthesis, the high-energy phosphate bonds thus formed being the major cellular mechanism for energy storage. In the uncoupled state, heat rather than ATP is produced.

The mechanism of uncoupling and the role of UCP 1 are fairly well understood (Fig. 2.3). During oxidation of fatty acid chains by the respiratory mitochondrial enzymes, hydrogen atoms are extruded from the inner mitochondrial matrix, creating an electromotive gradient for reentry into the inner matrix; in the coupled state, this reentry is linked to ATP synthase, providing the energy for ATP synthesis. In BAT mitochondria, uniquely, UCP 1, when activated by free fatty acids, provides a channel for hydrogen ion reentry to the inner mitochondrial matrix without the synthesis of ATP and with the release of energy as heat.

BAT also possesses type 2 deiodinase that converts intracellular thyroxine (T4) into the physiologically active triiodothyronine (T3). This deiodinase is stimulated by NE (α_1 receptor). The increased T3 is essential for the full expression of UCP 1. Hypothyroidism, therefore, is associated with markedly diminished BAT thermogenesis. Heat production is regulated by NE, but T3 plays a permissive role.

SNS also regulates the growth of BAT in the cold and is responsible for cold acclimation, as discussed in subsequent sections.

"Beige" Adipocytes

In addition to the classic BAT described earlier, which is located in rather discrete masses in the interscapular and supraclavicular areas, evidence has emerged that adipocytes that share many of the features of the classic brown adipocytes can develop in white adipocyte tissue (WAT) depots, and perhaps skeletal muscle, by a process referred to as "browning." These beige adipocytes, furthermore, express UCP 1 and can be recruited by cold exposure and SNS stimulation. Several transcription factors that appear to regulate the development of beige adipocytes in WAT depots have been described. Because cold can induce the appearance of BAT in humans, the possibility that some of these BAT depots in adult humans may be composed largely of beige adipocytes has been raised. Research in the recruitment of functional BAT that would increase energy expenditure is of strong interest as a potential treatment for obesity. This is a rapidly evolving field that holds the promise of identifying targets for drug development.

TABLE 2.4	**SA Effects on Visceral Smooth Muscle**
Gastrointestinal tract $\downarrow$ motility (α_1-, α_2-, β_1-, β_2-mediated relaxation) $\uparrow$ sphincter tone (α_1)	
Urinary bladder $\downarrow$ motility (β_2 relaxation) $\uparrow$ sphincter and trigone (α_1)	
Uterus $\downarrow$ motility (β_2 relaxation)	
Bronchial musculature $\downarrow$ tone (β_2-mediated relaxation)	

SA, sympathoadrenal.

Sympathoadrenal Effects on Visceral Smooth Muscle and Exocrine Glands

The routine functioning of the GI tract and urinary bladder is under the principal control of the parasympathetic nervous system that stimulates contraction of the gut and increases gut motility. The "enteric nervous system" consisting of the plexuses of Meissner and Auerbach, located in the submucosa and intramuscular regions of the GI tract, receives both a parasympathetic and sympathetic innervation and mediates relaxation of the visceral smooth muscle via intestinal neuropeptides and nitric oxide.

Gastrointestinal, urinary tract, and bronchial smooth muscle inhibition

As would be expected as part of the "fight or flight" response, SA stimulation decreases both the motility and the exocrine secretion of the GI tract. The effects are mediated principally by the β_2 receptor (motility) and the α_2 receptor (glandular secretion). Part of the suppression of GI activity is the stimulation, via the α_1 receptor, of the GI sphincters (Table 2.4).

The detrusor muscle of the bladder is also relaxed (β_2 mediated) and the corresponding sphincter contracted (α_1). Uterine and bronchial smooth muscle are relaxed as well (β_2 mediated).

Sympathoadrenal Effects on Renal Function, Electrolytes, and Hormone Secretion

Sympathetic nervous system effects on the kidney

The renal vasculature, the juxtaglomerular apparatus, and the renal tubules are all innervated by the SNS, and all three areas play a role in the regulation of blood volume, blood pressure, and sodium excretion (Table 2.5). Stimulation of the

TABLE 2.5	**SNS Effects on the Kidney**
Vasoconstriction	
Decrease renal blood flow and GFR	
Shunts blood from the cortical to the juxtamedullary nephrons	
Increases sodium reabsorption	
Direct α_1-mediated effect on renal tubule	
Stimulation of renin release	
β_1-mediated effect on juxtaglomerular cells	
Increased A II and aldosterone production	

GFR, glomerular filtration rate; SNS, sympathetic nervous system; A II, angiotensin II.

vasculature (α_1 mediated) decreases renal blood flow and glomerular filtration rate, and NE at the juxtaglomerular cells increases renin release (β_1 mediated), whereas a direct effect on the renal tubular epithelium (α_1 mediated) increases sodium and water reabsorption.

The enhanced renal sodium reabsorption, therefore, has both direct and indirect components, all of which reinforce each other. SNS stimulation of renin secretion activates the renin–angiotensin–aldosterone system (RAAS), thereby enhancing distal tubular sodium reabsorption. Renal arteriolar vasoconstriction preferentially shunts blood from the superficial cortical to the deeper juxtaglomerular nephrons with longer loops that are more efficient at sodium reabsorption. The net result is a substantial increase in renal avidity for sodium.

DA that is generated in the renal tubules from circulating DOPA increases sodium excretion by the kidneys.

Effect on serum potassium and phosphate

Catecholamines alter the cellular uptake of potassium in a complicated fashion that affects the serum level: α receptor stimulation increases and β receptor activation decreases the circulating levels of potassium. In general, the β receptor effect predominates so that catecholamines decrease and β blockers increase serum potassium.

E has been shown to lower serum phosphate by a β_2 receptor mechanism. This is the likely explanation for the hypophosphatemia noted in situations of marked SA activation such as myocardial infarction.

Sympathoadrenal effects on endocrine glands and hormone secretion

Many endocrine glands possess adrenergic receptors and receive a sympathetic innervation. SA effects operate outside of the usual feedback loops that normally regulate hormone secretion, and in general these feedback loops supersede the SA effects. SA stimulation of thyroid and parathyroid hormone release may be seen as reinforcements for "fight or flight," assuring availability of calcium as an important downstream activator of catecholamine effects (PTH) and amplifying the effects of catecholamines on the heart (thyroid).

Of greater importance in physiologic regulation are the effects on renin and insulin. As noted earlier, renin release activates the RAAS and contributes to sodium conservation; additionally, the angiotensin II so generated increases BP and directs blood flow to exercising muscle, the later served by vessels dilated by locally produced vasodilator substances such as lactate. The increased angiotensin II also stimulates central SNS outflow.

Less well appreciated, but also very important, are the effects of the SNS on insulin secretion. The pancreatic β cells are well endowed with sympathetic nerve endings and with both α and β receptors; the β_2 receptor increases, whereas the α_2 receptor suppresses insulin release. As is typical of tissues possessing both receptor types, the β receptor predominates at low agonist levels, whereas the α receptor is dominant at higher NE concentrations, as occurs with intense SNS stimulation. α-mediated suppression is the clinically relevant effect in situations of marked SA activation. In patients with pheochromocytoma, for example, impaired glucose tolerance or frank diabetes mellitus is "cured" by α blockade prior to surgery, an effect associated with marked increase in insulin levels. Suppression of insulin also contributes importantly to the ketoacidosis described in subsequent sections.

BIBLIOGRAPHY BY CATEGORY

GENERAL

Young JB, Landsberg L. Physiology of the sympathoadrenal system (Chapter 13). In: Wilson JD, Foster DW, Kronenberg HM, et al., eds. *Williams Textbook of Endocrinology.* 9th ed. Philadelphia: WB Saunders; 1998.

BAT

Bartness TJ, Vaughan CH, Song CK. Sympathetic and sensory innervation of brown adipose tissue. *Int J Obes.* 2010;34:S36–S42.

Enerbäck S. Brown adipose tissue in humans. *Int J Obes.* 2010;34;S43–S46.

Kajimura S. Promoting brown and beige adipocyte biogenesis through the PRDM16 pathway. *Int J Obes Suppl.* 2015;5:S11–S14.

Kajimara S, Seale P, Spiegelman BM. Transcriptional control of brown fat development. *Cell Metab.* 2010;11:257–262.

Morrison SF, Madden CJ, Tupone D. Central control of brown adipose tissue thermogenesis. *Front Endocrinol.* 2012;3:1–19.

Muzik O, Manger TJ, Granneman JG. Assessment of oxidative metabolism in brown fat using PET imaging. *Front Endocrinol.* 2012;3:1–7.

Ricquier D. Uncoupling protein 1 of brown adipocytes, the only uncoupler: a historical perspective. *Front Endocrinol.* 2011,2:1–7.

Rosenbaum M, Leibel RL. Adaptive thermogenesis in humans. *Int J Obes.* 2010;34:S47–S55.

Tchernof A, Richard D. Physiological determinants and impacts of the adipocyte phenotype. *Int J Obes Suppl.* 2015;5:S21–S22.

Townsend KL, Tseng Y-H. Of mice and men: novel insights regarding constitutive and recruitable brown adipocytes. *Int J Obes Suppl.* 2015;5:S15–S20.

Yoneshiro T, Aita S, Matsushita M, et al. Brown adipose tissue, whole-body energy expenditure, and thermogenesis in health adult men. *Obesity.* 2011;19:13–16.

LIPOLYSIS

Coppack SW, Jensen MD, Miles JM. In vivo regulation of lipolysis in humans. *J Lipid Res.* 1994;35:177–186.

REGULATION OF GLYCOGENOLYSIS

Cohen P. The origins of protein phosphorylation. *Nat Cell Biol.* 2002;4:E127–E130.

Reitman ML. FGF21: a missing link in the biology of fasting. *Cell Metab.* 2007;5:405–407.

RENAL FUNCTION

Bello-Reuss E, Trevino DL, Gottschalk CW. Effect of renal sympathetic nerve stimulation on proximal water and sodium reabsorption. *J Clin Invest.* 1976;57:1104–1107.

Dibona GF, Kopp UC. Neural control of renal function. *Physiol Rev.* 1997;1:75–197.

Gill Jr JR, Casper AGT. Role of the sympathetic nervous system in the renal response to hemorrhage. *J Clin Invest.* 1969;48:915–922.

THERMOGENESIS

Girardier L, Stock MJ, eds. *Mammalian Thermogenesis.* New York: Chapman and Hall; 1983.

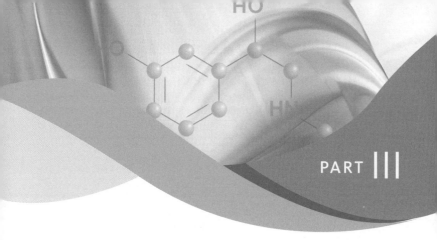

The Role of the
Sympathoadrenal System in Physiologic Adaptation and the Pathophysiology of Disease States

The SA system is essential for adaptation to external and internal threats that challenge the constancy of the internal environment. The SA effects are manifold combining direct effects on adrenergic receptors with coordinated changes in blood flow and hormone secretion.

Cold Exposure

Survival in the cold was a critical development in the evolution of mammals. The integrated response to cold exposure includes heat generation and heat conservation dependent upon SA regulation of metabolism and the cardiovascular system. Both the SNS and the adrenal medulla are involved with the SNS playing the dominant role. Temperature-sensing neurons in the hypothalamus, brainstem and spinal cord, as well as in the skin, initiate the SA response to a fall in temperature. SNS activation in the cold is shown in Figure 1.15 in laboratory rodents for heart; similar changes occur in BAT.

Heat conservation

Peripheral arterial and superficial venous constriction limits blood flow to the skin diminishing heat loss and improving the insulating capacity of the subcutaneous tissues. Venoconstriction is most marked in the superficial veins of the extremities which are endowed with more α_2 adrenergic receptors than the deep veins where α_1 receptors predominate. As external cooling decreases the affinity of the venous α_1 receptors (deep veins) to NE while, conversely, increasing the affinity for NE on the α_2 receptors (superficial veins), cold exposure shifts blood to the deep venous system. Increased blood flow to the deep veins of the limbs, which forms a plexus around the arteries, increases the efficiency of the countercurrent mechanism that removes heat from the arterial circulation and returns it to the central venous system. The circulation to the limbs thus plays a significant role in both heat conservation and heat loss.

Heat generation: nonshivering thermogenesis and cold acclimation

Shivering thermogenesis refers to the heat produced by muscular contractions induced by cold exposure. Shivering is mediated by the somatic nervous system but is apparently facilitated by catecholamines. In fur-bearing mammals, piloerection provides insulation; in humans, this has little effect on heat conservation but produces well-recognized "goose pimples" or "goose bumps." Piloerection is mediated by the α_1 receptor.

Nonshivering thermogenesis (NST) refers to metabolic heat production in response to cold exposure. It has been studied extensively in laboratory rodents. BAT is the origin of the heat produced. The SNS turns on heat production via the β_3 adrenergic receptor as described in the previous section. The SNS also drives the hypertrophy of BAT that accompanies cold acclimation. Cold acclimation, which occurs after prolonged exposure to cold, greatly potentiates heat production in BAT (Fig. 3.1), a consequence of the enlarged mass of BAT and the important fact that tachyphylaxis does not occur with prolonged stimulation as the β_3 receptor, unlike other β receptors, does not undergo desensitization. Cold acclimation in fact is defined by an enhanced thermogenic response to NE.

Although generally recognized as a significant physiologic process in humans at present, the concept of regulated production of metabolic heat in large adult mammals has had a checkered history and was commonly regarded with skepticism until the 1970s. The issue was settled by experiments on army recruits who, after prolonged cold exposure, stopped shivering and increased metabolic rate, thus demonstrating that cold acclimation and NST had occurred. The site of origin of NST in humans remained controversial until the last decade when functioning BAT was unequivocally demonstrated by positon emission tomography scans, biopsy, and the demonstration of UCP 1 in fat depots identified in imaging studies.

The anatomic location of BAT, adjacent to the great vessels, and the vascularity of BAT maximize distribution of the heat throughout the body.

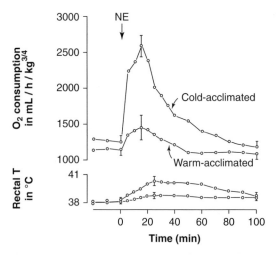

FIGURE 3.1. NE-stimulated thermogenesis in the rat: effect of cold acclimation. NE increases oxygen consumption (and rectal temperature), in both cold-acclimated (*closed circle*) and warm-acclimated (*open circle*) curarized rats. The effect is markedly enhanced in cold-acclimated animals; it is the hallmark of cold acclimation. NE, norepinephrine. (From Hseih ACL, Carlson LD, Gray G. Role of the sympathetic nervous system in the control of chemical regulation of heat production. *Am J Physiol.* 1957;190:247–251.)

Cardiovascular changes in cold exposure

In addition to the vasoconstrictive changed induced by the SNS during heat conservation as described above, cardiac stimulation driven by the SNS increases cardiac output. This serves the function of distributing heat generated by NST and delivering substrates for metabolizing tissues throughout the body. In acute cold exposure, blood pressure is elevated but the rise in BP is not sustained.

Substrate mobilization in cold exposure

The SA system stimulates lipolysis and glycogenolysis during cold exposure both directly and by suppressing the release of insulin and stimulating the release of glucagon. SA activation of hormone-sensitive lipase, lipoprotein lipase, and stimulation of hepatic glucose output are involved in the response to cold exposure.

Exercise and Physical Training

As a critical component of the "fight or flight" response, it is no surprise that exercise is associated with significant SA activation (Fig. 3.2). The enhanced activity of the SNS and adrenal medulla originates in the conscious and

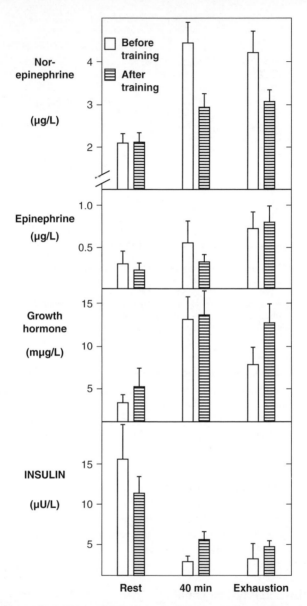

FIGURE 3.2. Plasma concentrations before and after training are compared at rest, at 40 minutes of exercise, and just before exhaustion. (From Hartley LH, Mason JW, Hogan RP, et al. Multiple hormonal responses to prolonged exercise in relation to physical training. *J Appl Physiol.* 1972;33:607–610.)

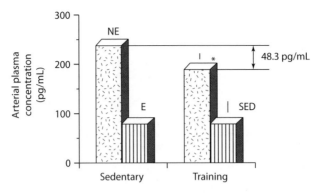

FIGURE 3.3. Bar graph shows the mean arterial plasma concentration of NE and epinephrine (E) for the sedentary and training phases. Plasma NE concentration was reduced by 48.3 pg per mL or 21% with training, whereas plasma E concentration remained unchanged. SED, standard error of the difference. NE, norepinephrine. (From Meredith IT, Friberg P, Jennings GL, et al. Exercise training lowers resting renal but not cardiac sympathetic activity in humans. *Hypertension.* 1991;18:575–582.)

autonomic portions of the CNS. SA outflow during exercise is further modulated by changes in circulating levels of hormones and substrates and by the physical and chemical properties of the blood such as temperature, tonicity, pH, and oxygen and carbon dioxide tension. The SA system response is designed to address three major requirements of strenuous exertion: (1) the provision of oxygen and metabolic substrates to contracting muscle; (2) the need to dissipate excess heat generated by muscle contraction; and (3) maintenance of an adequate plasma volume. Training decreases SNS activity both during exercise and at rest (Figs. 3.2 and 3.3).

Cardiovascular effects of the sympathoadrenal system in exercise

Cardiac output is increased by the inotropic and chronotropic effects of catecholamines on the heart and the increase in venous return that occurs with venoconstriction and with the increase in blood flow from exercising muscle. The splanchnic and renal circulations are constricted whereas flow to the heart and skeletal muscle is increased due in large measure to the buildup of vasodilator metabolites such as lactate (from glycogenolysis) and purine metabolites (derived from ATP). The BP rises, often substantially, assuring perfusion of muscle and heart. Plasma volume is defended in the presence of sweating and evaporative fluid loss by enhanced renal sodium reabsorption, a direct effect of the SNS and the stimulation of renin release with the consequent production of angiotensin II (A II) and aldosterone. Heat is dissipated by cutaneous vasodilation and eccrine sweating, the later mediated by cholinergic sympathetic nerves to the sweat glands.

Substrate mobilization

Activation of the SA system provides substrate to support the increased metabolism in skeletal and cardiac muscle. Both circulating epinephrine (E) and SNS activity participate in the increased production of free fatty acids (FFA) and glucose that occurs during exercise. Suppression of insulin release by the SNS plays an important role and reinforces the direct effects of catecholamines on mobilization of substrates from energy stores in adipose tissue, skeletal muscle, and liver. Stimulation of hormone-sensitive lipase in adipocytes results in the liberation of FFA and glycerol; activation of phosphorylase in liver provides glucose from glycogen while muscle phosphorylase produces glucose for local consumption in muscle and provides lactate which is added to the general circulation. Gluconeogenesis in liver utilizes the glycerol and lactate produced in adipose tissue and glycogen, respectively.

Dietary Intake: Fasting and Overfeeding

Dietary intake exerts important effects on SA activity. The underlying physiologic mechanisms have been well worked out. The activity of the adrenal medulla and the SNS, although coordinated, is not congruent during fasting.

Fasting results in suppressed sympathetic nervous system activity and slightly stimulated adrenal medullary activity

As fasting is associated with the mobilization of substrates from energy stored as triglycerides and glycogen, and from increased gluconeogenesis, all processes stimulated by catecholamines, it had been widely assumed that fasting was associated with increased SNS activity. This supposition was dispelled in the 1970s when experiments employing NE turnover techniques demonstrated unequivocally that fasting suppresses the SNS (Fig. 3.4), as shown by the line of lesser scope. This decrease in SNS activity occurs in humans as well as in laboratory rodents (Fig. 3.5). Although well established, this effect of fasting on the SNS is insufficiently appreciated. As shown in Fig. 3.5, in distinction to the stimulation of the SNS, adrenal medullary activity is mildly increased during a fast. The increase in E is small but significant and much different from the huge increase in E secretion that occurs during hypoglycemia.

Three questions immediately arise in light of these facts: (1) How are substrates mobilized during fasting? (2) What physiologic function is subserved by SNS suppression? (3) What are the signals that link the SNS and dietary intake?

1. Substrate mobilization depends heavily on the fall in insulin secretion that accompanies fasting. This decrease in circulating insulin in conjunction with the small rise in E stimulates lipolysis and hepatic glucose output. Fibroblast growth factor 21 has also been proposed to stimulate lipolysis during fasting but this effect is controversial.

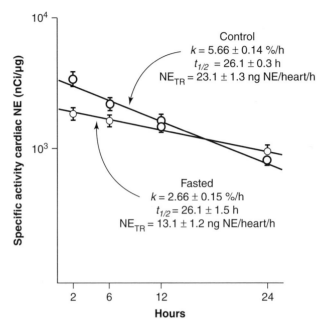

FIGURE 3.4. Fasting decreases NE turnover in heart. (Modified From Young JB, Landsberg L. Suppression of sympathetic nervous system during fasting. *Science.* 1977;196:1473–1475.)

2. Suppression of the SNS during fasting subserves the useful function of diminishing energy expenditure, a conservative mechanism that would prolong survival during fasting.
3. The physiologic mechanisms linking dietary intake with SNS activity have been well worked out: decreased insulin-mediated glucose uptake and metabolism in neurons of the ventromedial hypothalamus stimulates an inhibitory pathway to tonically active SNS neurons in the brainstem (Fig. 3.6). During fasting, the small fall in glucose and the larger fall in insulin decrease insulin-mediated glucose metabolism in the insulin-sensitive neurons of the ventromedial hypothalamus. This decrease in glucose metabolism stimulates an inhibitory pathway from the hypothalamus to the tonically active SNS neurons in the brainstem resulting in suppression of central sympathetic outflow. This is an example of regulation by descending inhibition, a fundamental principal elaborated by the famous British neurophysiologist Sir Charles Sherrington. Evidence for this sequence is summarized in Table 3.1.

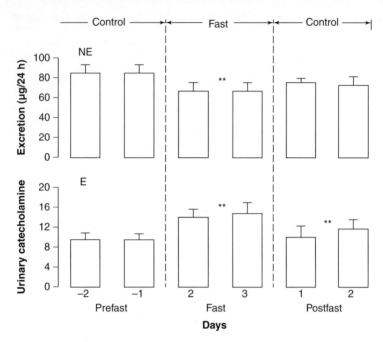

FIGURE 3.5. Effect of fasting on urinary catecholamine excretion in young, normal weight men. **$P < .001$. NE, norepinephrine; E, epinephrine. (From Young JB, Rosa RM, Landsberg L. Dissociation of sympathetic nervous system and adrenal medullary responses. *Am J Physiol.* 1984;247:E35–E40.)

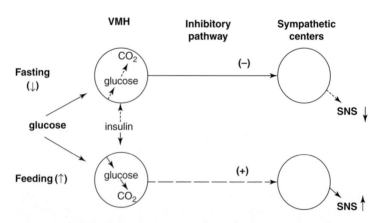

FIGURE 3.6. Model of dietary effects on SNS activity. (Modified From Young JB, Landsberg L. Impaired suppression of sympathetic activity during fasting in the gold thioglucose-treated mouse. *J Clin Invest.* 1980;65:1086–1094.)

TABLE 3.1	Insulin-Mediated Glucose Uptake in the VMH Regulates SNS Activity in Response to Diet

- Fasting suppresses the SNS
- Glucose stimulates the SNS
- Hypoglycemia suppresses the SNS
- 2-Deoxyglucose suppresses the SNS
  - Blocks intracellular glucose metabolism
- Insulin stimulates the SNS
- Gold thioglucose treatment (ablates the insulin glucose-sensitive VMH neurons) blocks the suppressive effect of fasting
  - SNS suppression with fasting is secondary to descending inhibition

VMH, ventromedial hypothalamus; SNS, sympathetic nervous system.

Feeding carbohydrates and fat, and overfeeding a mixed diet stimulates the sympathetic nervous system

In laboratory rodents, carbohydrates and fat added to the usual chow diet stimulates the SNS (Figs. 3.7 and 3.8). Dietary protein, in contrast, is without

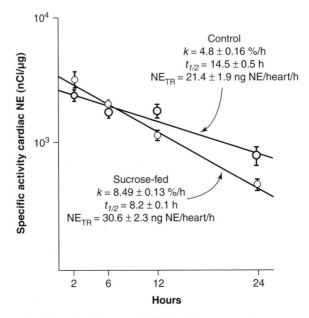

FIGURE 3.7.   Effect of sucrose on cardiac NE turnover. (From Young JB, Landsberg L. Stimulation of the sympathetic nervous system during sucrose feeding. *Nature.* 1977;269:615–617.)

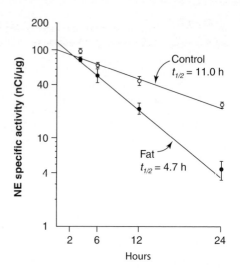

FIGURE 3.8. Effect of a fat-enriched diet on NE turnover in rat heart. Data are plotted as the means ± SEM for specific activity of hearts from four to six animals from each group at each time point. *Open circles* denote chow-fed rats (control), whereas *closed circles* represent fat-fed rats (control). The slope *k*, of each turnover line is significant at *P* < 0.0001. (From Schwartz JH, Young JB, Landsberg L. Effect of dietary fat on the sympathetic nervous system activity in the rat. *J Clin Invest.* 1983;72:361–370.)

effect even when added as excess calories (Fig. 3.9). Overfeeding a mixed ("cafeteria") diet also activates the SNS (Fig. 3.10). The link between diet and the SNS involves insulin and glucose and is the converse of that described above for fasting (Fig. 3.6). During feeding or overfeeding, the small rise in glucose and the large rise in insulin increases insulin-mediated glucose metabolism in the hypothalamic neurons thereby decreasing activity in the inhibitory pathway to the brainstem with release of the tonically active SNS neurons and an increase in central sympathetic outflow. These dietary effects occur in humans as well as in small mammals. The stimulatory effect of euglycemic insulin infusions on SNS activity in humans is shown in Figure 3.11.

Although the survival value of SNS suppression in the face of limits imposed on dietary intake is obvious in terms of decreased metabolic rate and conservation of fuel stores, the stimulatory effect of dietary excess on the SNS is less clear but is likely related to the metabolic adaptation to a low protein diet.

During the course of mammalian evolution, protein has been the limiting nutrient for growth and development, as pointed out by Harvard Professor George Cahill. The capacity to increase sympathetically mediated thermogenesis in the face of excess fat and carbohydrate would permit an organism on a subsistence diet deficient in essential nutrients to overeat the deficient diet, thereby fulfilling the requirements for the limiting nutrient (protein) while dissipating the excess calories as heat. The capacity to dissipate excess calories known as dietary thermogenesis, a mechanism entirely analogous to NST, would allow an organism to overeat and burn the extra calories rather than store them as fat. In this manner, dietary requirements for growth and development could be met without excess calorie storage as fat. Consistent with this interpretation is the fact that protein

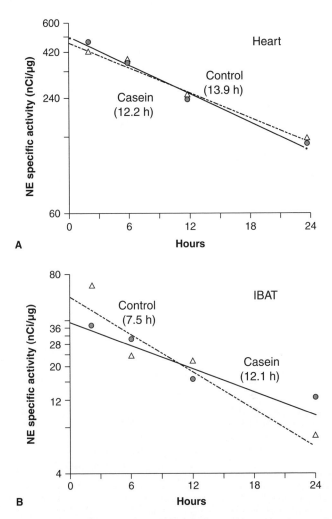

FIGURE 3.9.   No effect of casein on [³H]NE turnover in heart **(A)** and IBAT **(B)**. Animals were fed either a 2:1 mixture of chow and casein or chow alone for 5 days before the study. At the start of the turnover measurement, all rats received an intravenous injection of [³H]NE (100 µCi/kg) and were killed at various times over the ensuing 24 hours. In the figure, data are plotted as means for specific activity of NE in heart and IBAT from four to six animals in each group at each time point. *Closed circles* and the *solid line* represent rats given chow + casein; *open triangles* and the *broken line* represent animals given chow alone. The numbers in parentheses refer to the half-time disappearance of tracer ($t_{1/2}$). (From Kaufman LN, Young JB, Landsberg L. Effect of protein on sympathetic nervous system activity in the rat. Evidence for nutrient-specific responses. *J Clin Invest.* 1986;77:551–558.)

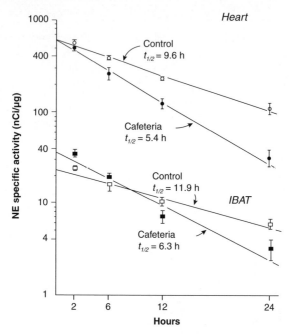

FIGURE 3.10.   Effect of overfeeding on NE turnover in heart and BAT. (Modified data from Young JB, Saville E, Rothwell NJ, et al. Effect of diet and cold exposure on norepinephrine turnover in brown adipose tissue of the rat. *J Clin Invest.* 1982;69:1061–1071.)

FIGURE 3.11.   Effect of insulin on SNS activity. **A:** (From Rowe JW, Young JB, Minaker KL, et al. Effect of insulin and glucose infusions on sympathetic nervous system activity in normal man. *Diabetes.* 1981;30(3):219–225.) **B:** (From Hausberg M, Mark AL, Hoffman RP, et al. Dissociation of sympathoexcitatory and vasodilator actions of modestly elevated plasma insulin levels. *J Hypertension.* 1995;13:1015–1021.)

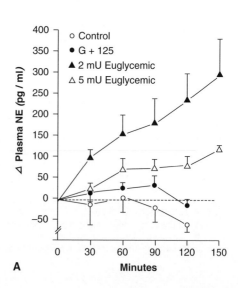

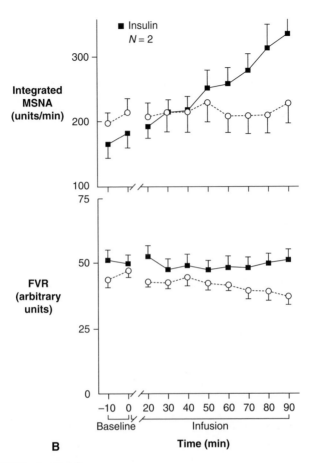

FIGURE 3.11. (*continued*)

does not stimulate the SNS (Fig. 3.9) and that low protein diets are extremely stimulatory (Fig. 3.12).

Hypoglycemia

In terms of cerebral metabolism, low glucose is equivalent to hypoxia; both oxygen and glucose are needed for normal brain function. When the plasma glucose falls below normal fasting levels, a series of hormonal (counter-regulatory) responses ensue in order to raise the blood sugar level toward normal.

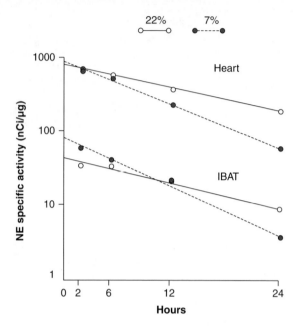

FIGURE 3.12.   Effect of 12 days of 7% protein feeding on [³H]NE turnover in rats. Open circles, rats fed 22% protein; closed circles, rats fed 7% protein. Feeding 7% protein increased NE turnover in heart and IBAT compared with 22% protein. (From Young JB, Kaufman LN, Saville ME, et al. Increased sympathetic nervous system activity in rats fed a low-protein diet. *Am J Physiol.* 1985;248:R627–R637.)

Glucose counter-regulation

E and glucagon are the principal counter-regulatory hormones. They both increase hepatic glucose output. In addition (Table 3.2), E stimulates lipolysis which provides alternative substrates (FFA) for use in tissues such as muscle, thereby sparing glucose for the brain, which requires glucose. E also suppresses endogenous insulin release by an α adrenergic effect on the pancreatic β cells, and inhibits insulin-mediated glucose uptake in muscle, thereby increasing glucose availability for the brain (Table 3.2).

Hypoglycemia is sensed in the ventromedial hypothalamus as well as in other areas of the brainstem. These glucose-sensitive neurons stimulate E secretion from the adrenal medulla (Fig. 3.13). Hypoglycemia, as noted above, suppresses the SNS; the rise in plasma NE, that accompanies the much larger rise in E, originates from the adrenal medulla (Fig. 3.13). E levels gradually increase as the blood sugar falls within the normal range (90 to 65 mg per dL). At levels below 50 mg per dL, the increase in adrenal medullary E is particularly intense, increasing 25 to 50 times baseline.

TABLE 3.2	Counter-Regulatory Effects of Epinephrine

- Increases glucose production
  - Glycogenolysis and gluconeogenesis in liver
  - Stimulation of glucose production from lactate derived from skeletal muscle (Cori cycle)
- Increases in lipolysis
  - Provision of alternative substrates (free fatty acids) for tissues outside the brain
- Inhibits insulin-mediated glucose uptake in skeletal muscle
  - Increases glucose availability for the brain
- Suppresses endogenous insulin release
  - Direct effect on pancreatic β cells
- Hypoglycemia awareness
  - Tremor, palpitations, anxiety → food-seeking behavior

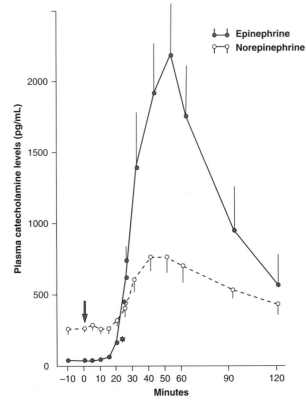

FIGURE 3.13. Effect of insulin-induced hypoglycemia on plasma epinephrine and norepinephrine levels. After an intravenous injection of 0.15 units per kg of regular insulin at time 0, plasma levels of epinephrine rise 50-fold in normal human subjects. (Reproduced from Garber AJ, et al. The role of adrenergic mechanisms in the substrate and hormonal response to insulin-induced hypoglycemia in man. *J Clin Invest.* 1976;58:7–15, by copyright permission of The American Society for Clinical Investigation.)

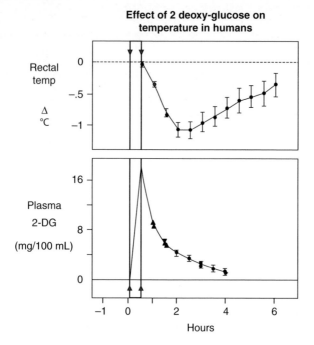

Effect of 2 deoxy-glucose on temperature in humans

FIGURE 3.14.   Effect of 2 DG on rectal temperature. (From Freinkel N, Metzger BE, Harris E, et al. The hypothermia of hypoglycemia. Studies with 2-deoxy-D-glucose in normal human subjects and mice. *N Engl J Med.* 1972;287:841.)

In addition to the provision of glucose, E secretion during hypoglycemia provokes tachycardia, increased pulse pressure, tremor, and anxiety. These adrenergic symptoms constitute an early warning system that alerts the subject to the development of hypoglycemia. Profuse sweating (eccrine rather than adrenergic) also occurs mediated not by E but rather by cholinergic sympathetic nerves. The sweating is induced by the fall in temperature set point that accompanies acute hypoglycemia (Fig. 3.14); the sweating is the mechanism that induces the fall in temperature to meet the new temperature set point.

Hypoglycemia unawareness in diabetics

Although both E and glucagon are involved in the counter-regulatory response in normal individuals, an adequate counter-regulatory response (recovery from hypoglycemia) occurs with either E or glucagon alone in the absence of the other. In insulin-dependent diabetics, however, glucagon response to hypoglycemia typically fails after about 5 years of insulin deficiency, leaving E as the sole acute defense against hypoglycemia. The reasons for this failure of the glucagon response are not entirely clear and probably multifactorial, but the absence of insulin within the pancreatic islets likely plays a major role as it is known that intra-islet insulin is required for a normal glucagon counter-regulatory response.

Should the E response fail, therefore, diabetic patients would be at risk of severe hypoglycemic attacks. Unfortunately, it is not uncommon for the E response to fail in long-standing diabetics. The impact of this failure is twofold: (1) the typical adrenergic warning signs of hypoglycemia, dependent as they are on adrenal medullary E, are absent; and (2) in the absence of both glucagon and E, restoration of the plasma glucose does not occur. The consequence is severe, often devastating, hypoglycemia that occurs without warning.

The reasons for the failure of the adrenal medullary response in long-standing diabetics appear to be antecedent episodes of iatrogenic hypoglycemia giving rise to the designation "hypoglycemia-associated autonomic failure." The adrenal medullary response can be restored by prolonged periods of glucose control with studious avoidance of hypoglycemia.

Ketosis, Ketogenesis, and Ketoacidosis

The SA system plays an important role in the generation of ketones and in the development of ketoacidosis. The balance between insulin and catecholamines is the major determinant of ketoacidosis; this reciprocal relationship is nowhere better demonstrated than in the pathogenesis of ketosis. It is well recognized that low to absent levels of insulin are essential for the formation of ketone bodies in the liver. It is also known that the delivery of FFA to the liver provides the substrate for ketone formation and that FFA availability is the rate-limiting step in hepatic ketone formation. It is less well appreciated that catecholamine-induced lipolysis plays a major role in ketogenesis by increasing the flux of FFA to the liver. It is generally unrecognized that catecholamine-induced suppression of insulin release is a critical determinant in the pathogenesis of ketoacidosis in several clinical situations as outlined below.

In situations associated with ketosis, carbohydrate-derived Krebs cycle substrates are depleted, from starvation or diabetes, and acetyl CoA synthesis is increased from the flow of FFA to the liver. The buildup of acetyl CoA results in ketone body formation; in the presence of low insulin lipogenesis is impaired and entrance into the Krebs cycle is limited. When the liver is in this ketogenic mode, FFA delivery to the liver determines the rate of ketoacid formation; FFA delivery depends upon the relative balance of insulin and catecholamines which determines the extent of lipolysis. Glucagon may also stimulate lipolysis in the insulin-deficient state but is not essential for ketogenesis.

Starvation ketosis

Ketosis in starvation is characteristically mild and not associated with significant ketoacidosis as insulin levels are low but not absent, and E levels are increased but not markedly so. Under these circumstances, lipolysis is increased, but the flow of FFA to the liver is relatively restrained, limiting ketoacid production to a level short of that needed to produce frank acidosis. In clinical situations associated with increased carbohydrate requirements, however, a state of "accelerated" starvation may result in ketoacidosis as pointed out by Northwestern professor Norbert Freinkel decades ago. These situations include infancy, pregnancy, lactation, and hyperthyroidism.

Alcoholic ketoacidosis

Ketoacidosis occurs after a sustained drinking binge in nutritionally (glycogen) depleted chronic alcoholics. The characteristic picture is one of severe volume depletion due to vomiting and diarrhea. The SA system is markedly stimulated resulting in unrestrained lipolysis (β receptor mediated) and, most importantly, suppressed insulin release (α mediated). The complete suppression of insulin is what distinguishes alcoholic ketoacidosis from simple starvation. The importance of volume depletion is validated by the prompt response to volume resuscitation which relives the restraint on insulin secretion and corrects the acidosis without the administration of insulin, as well as the occurrence of ketoacidosis in other situations of extreme volume depletion such as *hyperemesis gravidarum*.

Diabetic ketoacidosis

Diabetic ketoacidosis occurs predominantly in type 1 diabetics where the absence of insulin is virtually complete. Ketoacidosis develops when therapeutic insulin is omitted, resulting in glycosuria, volume depletion, and unrestrained lipolysis. In type 2 diabetics, the low, but not absent, level of insulin is enough to blunt the lipolytic response so that glycosuria and hypertonicity dominate the clinical picture without ketoacidosis, although in the face of extreme volume depletion, SNS suppression of insulin may result in significant ketosis and ketoacidosis, which remits with adequate treatment.

Hypertension

Sympathetic nervous system activity in patients with essential hypertension

Until relatively recently, the SNS was not considered a major factor in the pathogenesis of essential hypertension. Even a casual analysis, though, had made it abundantly clear that the SNS played at least a permissive role in maintaining high BP as the sympathetic reflexes that made upright posture possible were normally active in hypertensive subjects and as adrenergic blockers lowered BP. Once adequate methods for the assessment of SNS activity were developed, full appreciation of the role played by catecholamines in the pathogenesis of hypertension was possible. The recent application of a variety of techniques has demonstrated decisively that SNS activity is increased in subjects with essential

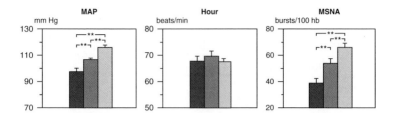

FIGURE 3.15. Mean arterial pressure (MAP) and MSNA in controls, mild and severe hypertension. (From Mancia G, Grassi G, Giannattasio C, et al. Sympathetic activation in the pathogenesis of hypertension and progression of organ damage. *Hypertension.* 1999;34(4, pt 2):724–748.)

hypertension. The increase in SNS activity, moreover, is greater in patients with more severe hypertension (Fig. 3.15). The SNS, therefore, plays a major role in the initiation and maintenance of high BP.

Effects of sympathetic nervous system activation on blood pressure

Stimulation of the heart, the veins, the kidneys, and the arterioles all contribute to the increase in BP that occurs with an increase in sympathetic tone (Fig. 2.1). The two physiologic components of an increase in BP, cardiac output and peripheral resistance, are both influenced by the SNS: cardiac output is increased by enhanced cardiac contractility and augmented venous return, the latter by venoconstriction and increased renal sodium reabsorption. Peripheral resistance is increased by arteriolar vasoconstriction mediated by direct SNS stimulation (α receptors) and by A II secondary to sympathetic stimulation of renin release (β receptors). These interrelationships are shown in Fig. 2.1.

Renal sympathetic nervous system activity and the pressure natriuresis relationship

The net effect of SNS stimulation of the kidney is to increase renal sodium reabsorption (Table 2.5). This is mediated by a direct effect on renal tubular epithelium, by renin release with the generation of A II and downstream stimulation of aldosterone secretion, and by renal vasoconstriction, stimulated directly by NE and A II. By its effect on renal sodium reabsorption, SNS stimulation of the kidney is one of the factors that alters the pressure natriuresis relationship, a necessary precondition for the development of sustained hypertension.

As pointed out by Professor Arthur Guyton of the University of Mississippi decades ago, the kidney has an infinite capacity to lower BP by increasing sodium (and hence water) excretion. As the perfusion pressure rises, sodium excretion also increases, counteracting the increase in pressure at the expense of the extracellular fluid volume. In order for sustained hypertension to develop,

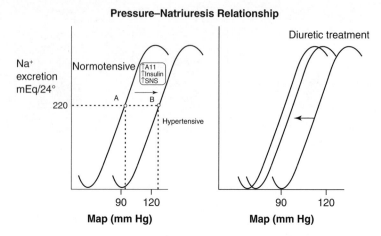

FIGURE 3.16.   (From Landsberg L. *On Rounds: 1000 Internal Medicine Pearls.* Philadelphia, PA: Wolters Kluwer; 2016.)

this normal relationship has to be reset, implying that any hypertensive state is associated with an abnormal pressure natriuresis relationship, the latter reflective of an increased renal avidity for sodium. This relationship, shown in Fig. 3.16, has been validated in numerous experimental studies. The important point here is that renal avidity for sodium is the *sine qua non* for the development of a sustained increase in BP. SNS activity is one factor increasing that avidity and driving the pressure natriuresis relationship to the right.

Viewed in these terms, hypertension may be seen as a compensatory mechanism for the increased renal avidity for sodium. Extracellular fluid volume, unlike BP, is closely regulated; a small mismatch in sodium intake and excretion has important physiologic consequences (volume overload or shock) whereas BP varies widely throughout the 24-hour cycle without adverse consequences. A higher BP, therefore, restores sodium balance and maintains extracellular fluid volume by overcoming the enhanced renal sodium reabsorption. The short-term problems attendant on fluid overload are thus avoided. Like any compensatory mechanism, however, there is a price to pay; in this case, the long-term cardiovascular risk associated with high BP.

The pressure natriuresis relationship also explains why all diuretics, independent of class or mechanism of action, are effective treatments of hypertension. By helping the kidneys excrete salt, the pressure natriuresis relationship is restored toward normal (Fig. 3.16).

There is an evolutionary aspect underlying both the enhanced SNS activity and renal avidity for sodium. For these traits to have persisted throughout the course of human evolution they must have had survival value. Enhanced SNS activity and increased renal avidity for sodium are traits that would provide protection from volume depletion or hemorrhage, thereby improving the chances of survival in the face of challenges imposed by the external environment. The long-term consequences of these traits, such as hypertension, would be played out over years, usually past reproductive age and therefore not selected against by evolutionary pressure.

Obesity

Sympathetic activity in obesity

Up until the mid-1980s conventional wisdom held that SNS activity was reduced in obesity. This erroneous belief was based on the fact that heritable forms of rodent obesity such as the *ob/ob* mouse had reduced SNS activity, and on the fact that SNS activity increased metabolic rate. It was thus supposed that a decrease in SNS activity contributed to the obese state by decreasing metabolism. It is now well recognized that the usual forms of obesity are, on the contrary, associated with increased SNS activity (Figs. 3.17 and 3.18).

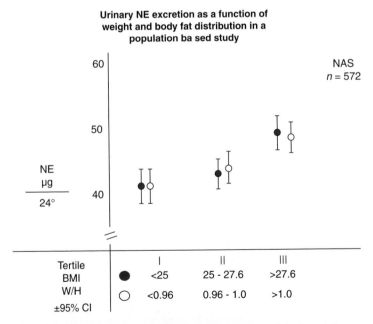

FIGURE 3.17. (From Troisi RJ, Weiss ST, Parker DR, et al. Relation of obesity and diet to sympathetic nervous system activity. *Hypertension.* 1991;17:669–677.)

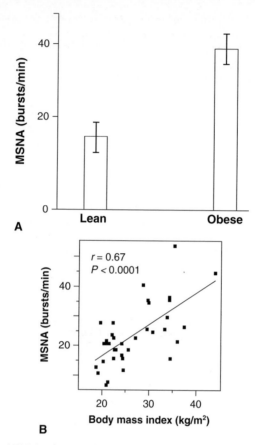

FIGURE 3.18.   MSNA in relation to obesity. **A:** (From Vollenweider P, Randin B, Tappy L, et al. Impaired insulin-induced sympathetic neural activation and vasodilation in skeletal muscle in obese humans. *J Clin Invest.* 1994;93:2365–2371.) **B:** (From Scherrer U, Randin B, Tappy L, et al. Body fat and sympathetic nerve activity in healthy subjects. *Circulation.* 1994;89:2634–2540.)

The increased SNS activity is caused by insulin (Fig. 3.11) and leptin. Leptin, the polypeptide product of the *ob/ob* gene, is produced by adipocytes; it depresses appetite and stimulates the SNS, thus increasing energy expenditure. It is deficient in the *ob/ob* mouse and in a rare familial form of human obesity but increased in the usual cases of human obesity. Leptin, along with insulin, which is elevated in the obese because of insulin resistance, stimulates central sympathetic outflow. With weight loss, which lowers both insulin and leptin, SNS activity decreases (Fig. 3.19) as does BP.

The increased SNS activity in the obese may be seen as a compensatory mechanism recruited in the obese to increase metabolic rate and restore energy balance

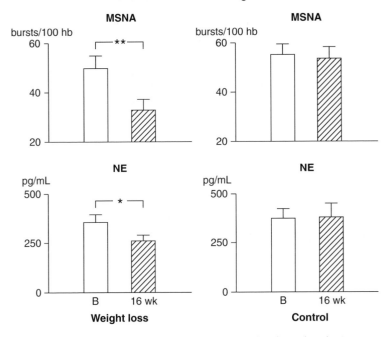

**Muscle sympathetic nervous activity (MSNA) before
and after 16 weeks of weight loss**

FIGURE 3.19. (From Grassi G, Seravalle G, Colombo M, et al. Body weight reduction, sympathetic nerve traffic, and arterial baroreflex in obese normotensive humans. *Circulation.* 1998; 97:2037–2042.)

(Fig. 3.20). An increase in BP is the unwanted consequence of this compensatory mechanism.

Adrenal medullary activity in obesity

In distinction to the SNS, the adrenal medulla is suppressed in the obese (Fig. 3.21). The lower levels of E are associated with the characteristic lipid abnormalities found in obesity: low high-density lipoprotein (HDL)-cholesterol and high triglycerides (Fig. 3.22). Interestingly, these same changes are seen in patients treated with β-blocking agents, implying that they are the consequence of antagonizing circulating E.

The metabolic syndrome

Abnormalities associated with obesity frequently form a cluster of traits that are known as the metabolic syndrome. Although the existence of this syndrome as a distinct entity has been questioned, there is little doubt that the

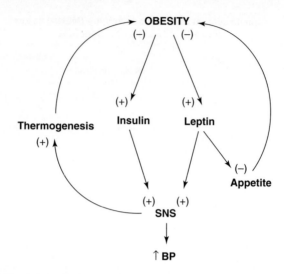

FIGURE 3.20.   Relationship between obesity and blood pressure. (From Landsberg L. Insulin-mediated sympathetic stimulation: role in the pathogenesis of obesity-related hypertension (or, how insulin affects blood pressure, and why). *J Hypertens.* 2001;19:523–528.)

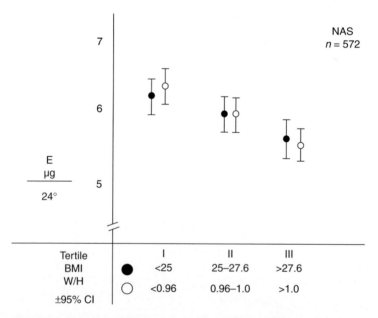

FIGURE 3.21.   (Modified from Landsberg L. Hyperinsulinemia: possible role in obesity-induced hypertension. *Hypertension.* 1992;19:161–166.)

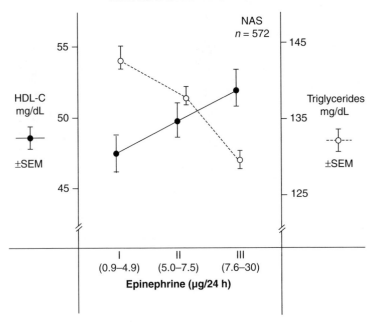

Epinephrine excretion, triglycerides and HDL-cholesterol levels in the NAS

NAS
n = 572

HDL-C
mg/dL

±SEM

Triglycerides
mg/dL

±SEM

I
(0.9–4.9)

II
(5.0–7.5)

III
(7.6–30)

Epinephrine (µg/24 h)

FIGURE 3.22   (Data from Ward KD, Sparrow D, Landsberg L, et al. The relationship of epinephrine excretion to serum lipid levels: The Normative Aging Study. *Metabolism*. 1994;43:509–513.)

principal components are more closely associated than could be accounted for by chance. The four cardinal features are: (1) the upper body form of obesity; (2) hypertension; (3) insulin resistance and consequent hyperinsulinemia; and (4) a characteristic dyslipidemia (low HDL-cholesterol and high triglycerides). Insulin resistance is the linchpin that ties the manifestations together (a better name would have been the "insulin resistance syndrome"). Insulin resistance and the upper body-abdominal form of obesity track together in both population based and clinical studies. Hyperinsulinemia develops in the face of insulin resistance as insulin release is stimulated by the increase in glucose that follows resistance to glucose uptake in skeletal muscle (the definition of insulin resistance). The hyperinsulinemia overcomes the block in glucose uptake but has adverse consequences: it stimulates the SNS, contributing to hypertension, and decreases E, which, along with hyperinsulinemia, contributes to the dyslipidemia (Fig. 3.22).

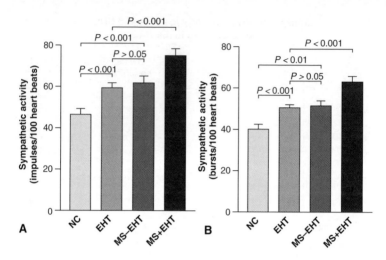

FIGURE 3.23.   MSNA in normal controls (NC), essential hypertension (EHT) in metabolic syndrome without hypertension (MS-HT) and in metabolic syndrome with hypertension (MS+HT). (From Huggett RJ, Burns J, Mackintosh AF, et al. Sympathetic neural activation in nondiabetic metabolic syndrome and its further augmentation by hypertension. *Hypertension.* 2004;44:847–852.)

Patients with the metabolic syndrome have increased SNS activity (Fig. 3.23), more pronounced in those with higher BP.

Hypoxia and Hypercarbia (Hypercapnia)

Lowered oxygen tension and increased partial pressure of carbon dioxide both increase SNS activity. These changes in the blood gases are sensed in the peripheral carotid and aortic bodies and central brainstem centers. The peripheral sensors are more important in the response to hypoxia, whereas the central receptors are critical for responding to hypercarbia. Decreased oxygen tension is sensed in the highly vascularized type I glomus cells of the carotid and aortic bodies and impulses sent via the IXth cranial nerve (carotid body) and the Xth cranial nerve (aortic body) to the nucleus of the solitary tract and thence to the SNS centers in the medulla that initiate changes in sympathetic outflow. Neurophysiologic studies demonstrate that the central processing of hypoxic and hypercapnic stimuli involves different pathways.

Chronic hypoxia

Chronic hypoxia in rats (Fig. 3.24) and humans (Fig. 3.25) is associated with a substantial increase in SNS activity. In humans at altitude, increased SNS

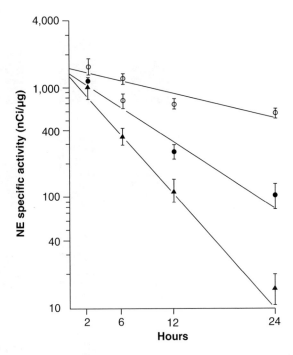

FIGURE 3.24.   Effect of two levels of chronic hypoxia on NE turnover in rat heart. Animals were maintained at 7.5% oxygen (severe hypoxia), 10.5% oxygen (moderate hypoxia), and 20.9% oxygen (control) for 7 days. *Open circle*, control (16.2 hours); *closed circle*, moderate hypoxia (6 hours); *filled triangle*, severe hypoxia (3.5 hours). (From Johnson TS, Young JB, Landsberg L. Sympathoadrenal responses to acute and chronic hypoxia in the rat. *J Clin Invest.* 1983;71:1263–1272.)

activity measured by muscle sympathetic nerve activity (MSNA) is associated with increased pulse rate, increased vascular resistance, and increased mean arterial pressure. Increases in adrenal medullary secretion may occur but are less consistent. The increase in SNS activity with hypoxia is not immediate; most studies indicate that in laboratory rodents and humans, acute hypoxia is associated with no change in sympathetic activity, or even a slight suppression. As would be expected from the effects of hypoxia and hypercarbia, patients with chronic respiratory failure have increased sympathetic activity and the increase is associated with increased morbidity and mortality (Fig. 3.26). Note that in distinction to the systemic vasoconstrictive effect the pulmonary vasoconstriction that accompanies hypoxia is not mediated by catecholamines, but rather by direct effects on ion channels in the pulmonary arterial tree.

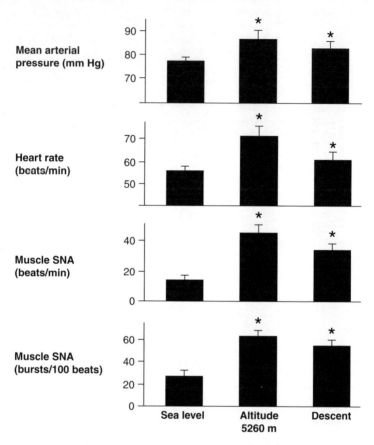

FIGURE 3.25.   Hemodynamic and sympathetic neural responses to high altitude acclimatization. Summary data (means ± SEM) for mean arterial pressure, heart rate, and muscle SNA during supine rest after 4 weeks at an altitude of 5,260 m, 3 days after return (descent), and 4 to 6 months after return from altitude (sea level). *$P < 0.05$ versus sea level; $n = 8$. (From Hansen J, Sander M. Sympathetic neural overactivity in healthy humans after prolonged exposure to hypobaric hypoxia. *J Physiol.* 2003;546(3):921–929.)

Obstructive sleep apnea

Obstructive sleep apnea (OSA) is associated with a significant increase in SNS activity (Fig. 3.27). Interestingly, the increased activity occurs during daytime wakefulness and not just during the disturbed sleep, and is associated with an increase in BP, making OSA a significant cause of secondary hypertension. Effective treatment decreases both the MSNA and the associated hypertension (Figs. 3.28 and 3.29).

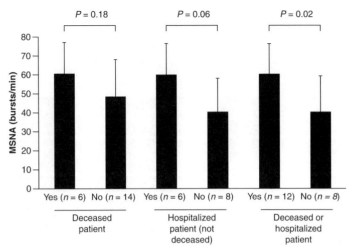

FIGURE 3.26. Association between MSNA and outcome in COPD patients. (From Andreas S, Haarmann H, Klarner S, et al. Increased sympathetic nerve activity in COPD is associated with morbidity and mortality. *Lung.* 2014;192(2):235–241.)

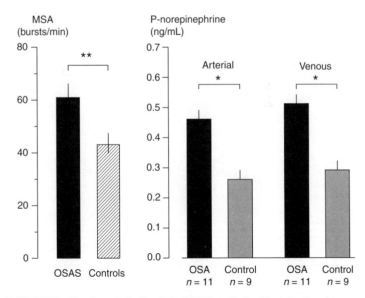

FIGURE 3.27. Muscle sympathetic activity (MSA) in patients with obstructive sleep apnea (OSA, $n = 11$) and controls ($n = 9$). Plasma concentration of norepinephrine (arterial and venous) in OSA patients (*filled bars*, $n = 11$) and controls (*shaded bars*). Shown are means $\pm$ SEM from 11 and 9 patients, respectively. *$P < 0.05$, **$P < 0.01$. (From Carlson JT, Hedner J, Elam M, et al. Augmented resting sympathetic activity in awake patients with obstructive sleep apnea. *Chest.* 1993;103:1763–1768.)

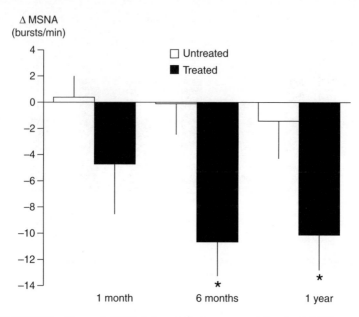

FIGURE 3.28. Changes in MSNA during repeated measurements in untreated OSA patients ($n = 9$) and in OSA patients treated with CPAP ($n = 11$). MSNA did not change in untreated patients. In treated patients, MSNA decreased after both 6 months and 1 year of CPAP treatment. *$P < 0.05$ versus baseline. (Data are mean ± SEM.) (From Narkiewicz K, Kato M, Phillips BG, et al. Nocturnal continuous positive airway pressure decreases daytime sympathetic traffic in obstructive sleep apnea. *Circulation.* 1999;100:2332–2335.)

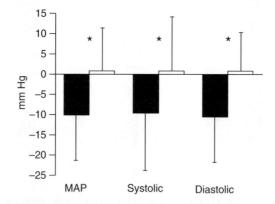

FIGURE 3.29. Changes in mean (MAP), systolic, and diastolic blood pressure with effective (*closed bars*) and subtherapeutic (*open bars*) CPAP. (*Asterisk*) Significant difference. (From Wolk R, Shamsuzzaman ASM, Somers VK. Obesity, sleep apnea, and hypertension. *Hypertension.* 2003;42:1067–1074.)

Congestive Heart Failure

An increase in sympathetic activity has been well documented in patients with congestive heart failure (CHF) (Figs. 3.30 and 3.31). Increased SNS activity may be viewed as a compensatory mechanism to increase cardiac output in the presence of a failing heart and to maintain blood flow to the brain and the heart

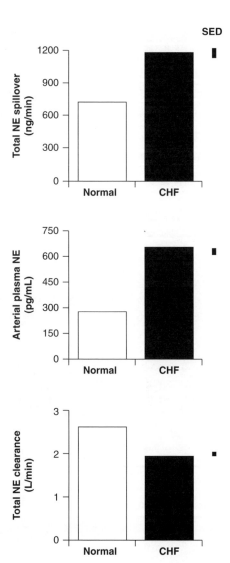

FIGURE 3.30. Bar graphs show total norepinephrine (NE) plasma kinetics in congestive heart failure (CHF) patients (*black bar*) and age-matched normal subjects (*white bars*). SED refers to the standard error of the difference (ANOVA). (From Meredith IT, Eisenhofer G, Lambert GW, et al. Cardiac sympathetic nervous activity in congestive heart failure. Evidence for increased neuronal norepinephrine release and preserved neuronal uptake. *Circulation.* 1993;88:136–145.)

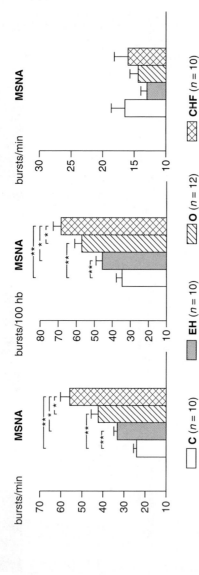

FIGURE 3.31. Sympathetic nerve activity to skeletal muscle (MSNA) and skin (SSNA) in control subjects (C) and in essential hypertensive (EH), obese (O), and congestive heart failure (CHF) patients. *$P < 0.05$, **$P < 0.01$. (From Grassi G, Colombo M, Seravalle G, et al. Dissociation between muscle and skin sympathetic nerve activity in essential hypertension, obesity, and congestive heart failure. *Hypertension.* 1998;31:64–67.)

TABLE 3.3	**The SNS in heart Failure**
The Heart	
Tachycardia $\rightarrow$ palpitations	
Increased contractile force $\rightarrow$ LVH	
Arrhythmias $\rightarrow$ palpitations, syncope, sudden death	
The Kidneys	
Vasoconstriction $\rightarrow$ $\downarrow$ GFR, $\downarrow$ RPF	
$\uparrow$ renin secretion $\rightarrow$ $\uparrow$ A II $\rightarrow$ $\uparrow$ aldosterone secretion $\rightarrow$ edema	
Dilutional hyponatremia	

GFR, glomerular filtration rate; SNS, sympathetic nervous system; LVH, left ventricular hypertrophy; A II, angiotensin II; RPF, renal plasma flow.

at the expense of other organs. The mechanisms responsible for the increased SNS activity in CHF are incompletely understood, but altered baroreceptor function appears to be involved. Unloading the pressure receptors in the carotid sinus, the aortic arch, and possibly the myocardium would decrease the restraint normally imposed on the tonically active SNS centers in the rostral ventrolateral medulla, resulting in increased SNS outflow.

The enhanced SNS tone contributes to some of the important clinical manifestations of CHF (Table 3.3), including tachycardia, increased force of contraction, left ventricular hypertrophy, and redistribution of blood flow from the kidneys and the gut. The increased SNS activity also increases sodium reabsorption, stimulates renin and thus A II formation, and constricts veins and arteries (excluding the brain and heart). Venoconstriction stiffens the veins diminishing compliance and giving rise to the physical sign known as "hepatojugular reflux." Compression of the right upper quadrant pushes blood into the nondistensible jugular veins which become visible in the neck. Renal vasoconstriction also decreases the glomerular filtration rate and the renal blood flow leading to prerenal azotemia and impairment in the ability of the kidney to sustain a water diuresis in the face of hypotonicity; coupled with the effects of A II to increase thirst, this impairment leads to hyponatremia.

Thyroid and Adrenal Hormones

Both thyroid and adrenal hormones have important interactions with catecholamines. The effects involve the activity of the SNS as well as the sensitivity of effector tissues to catecholamines (Fig. 3.32).

Effect of thyroid state on sympathetic nervous system activity

Although counterintuitive, hypothyroidism is associated with increased SNS activity. It seems reasonable that the increase in sympathetic activity is related to maintenance of body temperature via vasoconstriction (heat conservation) and metabolic heat generation, although the latter is compromised in the hypothyroid

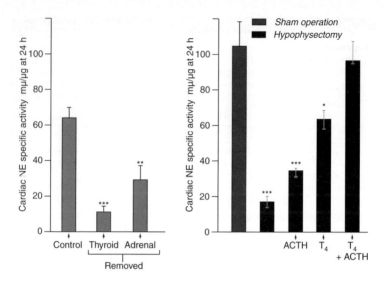

FIGURE 3.32. $*P < 0.05$, $**P < 0.01$, $***P < 0.001$. (From Landsberg L, Axelrod J. Influence of pituitary, thyroid, and adrenal hormones on norepinephrine turnover and metabolism in the rat heart. *Circ Res.* 1968;22:559–571.)

state. The sympathetically mediated increase in peripheral resistance is the cause of the hypertension frequently noted in hypothyroid patients.

Hyperthyroidism, on the other hand, is not associated with suppression of the SNS, despite the similarity of some of the effects of thyroid hormones and those of catecholamines, such as tachycardia and metabolic heat production.

Effect of thyroid state on sensitivity to catecholamines

It is commonly believed that β adrenergic responses are accentuated in the presence of thyroid hormone excess. Increases in the sensitivity to the physiologic effects of catecholamines, rigorously defined as changes in threshold or half maximal concentration for responses to β agonists, have, however, been difficult to demonstrate and many studies have produced contradictory results. Nonetheless, the "hyperadrenergic" manifestations of thyrotoxicosis, including tremor, stare, lid-lag, widened palpebral fissure, rapid reflex return, and anxiousness, are generally ameliorated by nonspecific β blockade.

In hypothyroidism, conversely, responsiveness to catecholamines may be diminished. Sympathetically mediated facultative NST, in particular, is impaired, as normal UCP function in BAT requires permissive amounts of triiodothyronine. Replacing thyroid hormone is essential for restoration of normal catecholamine responsiveness.

Effect of adrenal steroids on sympathetic nervous system activity and sensitivity

As in the case of hypothyroidism, deficiency of adrenal hormones is associated with enhanced SNS activity, and with decreased sensitivity to catecholamines. Normal responsiveness to catecholamines requires at least permissive amounts of glucocorticoids. The hypotension associated with adrenal insufficiency is characterized by inappropriate vasodilation; it is necessary to administer corticosteroids to restore normal responsiveness to sympathetic activity.

Hypotension and Shock

Dysfunction or suppression of the SNS plays a major role in many clinical situations associated with hypotension or shock. Neurologic diseases, drugs, or disordered sympathetic reflexes may all be involved in the pathogenesis of hypotensive reactions.

Orthostatic hypotension

Defined as a drop in BP of 20/10 mm Hg, usually with symptoms such as dizziness or, if severe enough, syncope, orthostatic hypotension occurs when the venous return falls substantially and the sympathetic reflexes that defend the BP cannot adequately compensate (Table 3.4). The usual causes are severe

TABLE 3.4 **Orthostatic Hypotension**
Fall in BP 20/30 mm Hg   Dizziness or syncope
Common causes   Dehydration; fluid loss; diuretics   Drugs that impair SNS function   Antihypertensives   Neuroleptics, antidepressants
Neurologic diseases of the SNS
Pure autonomic failure (idiopathic orthostatic hypotension)   Degeneration of the peripheral sympathetic nerves   Cause unknown
Multiple system atrophy (Shy–Drager)   Degeneration of the preganglionic cells of the interomediolateral cell column of the spinal cord   Widespread CNS degeneration (cerebellum; basal ganglia)   Cause unknown
Autoimmune autonomic neuropathy   Autoantibodies against the cholinergic nicotinic receptors of the preganglionic SNS neurons   May reflect prior infection (molecular mimicry) or paraneoplastic syndrome

BP, blood pressure; SNS, sympathetic nervous system; CNS, central nervous system.

volume depletion and/or impaired SNS response to the decreased venous return and the arterial hypotension. The latter may be the result of drugs that impair SNS function or specific diseases that affect the SNS. The drugs are typically antihypertensive medications or centrally acting agents that block sympathetic reflexes. The diseases include pure autonomic failure, autoimmune autonomic neuropathy, and **multiple system atrophy (MSA)**.

Previously called idiopathic orthostatic hypotension, **pure autonomic failure** is a degenerative disease of the peripheral (postganglionic) sympathetic nerves. The cause is unknown. Supine plasma levels of NE are low and do not increase with standing. The CNS is not involved but other manifestations of autonomic dysfunction such as dry eyes or genitourinary symptoms may occasionally develop.

MSA, also known as the Shy–Drager syndrome, is a sporadic, progressive, neuro-degenerative disease of the CNS that involves the basal ganglia, the cerebellum, and the autonomic nervous system. Parkinsonian features, cerebellar, or autonomic dysfunction may predominate. The intermediolateral cell column of the spinal cord that gives rise to the preganglionic sympathetic nerves degenerates, thereby interfering with the downward flow of impulses that engage the peripheral SNS. Failure of reflex baroreceptor activation is the result with attendant orthostatic hypotension; plasma NE fails to rise in response to upright posture.

Immunologic attack on the SNS is another cause of orthostatic hypotension. The so-called "autoimmune autonomic neuropathy" is associated with antibodies directed against the nicotinic cholinergic receptors in the sympathetic ganglia, thereby interrupting ganglionic transmission and blocking activation of the peripheral sympathetic nerves. The cause is unknown, but may be related to prior infection, and in some cases may be the result of a paraneoplastic syndrome.

Systemic diseases like amyloidosis and diabetes mellitus may also be associated with autonomic neuropathy.

Postural orthostatic tachycardia syndrome

A poorly understood syndrome of orthostatic intolerance, postural orthostatic tachycardia syndrome (POTS) is associated with tachycardia upon standing without an appreciable fall in BP. The cause is unknown but increased SNS activity on standing ("hyperadrenergic POTS"), decreased NE uptake in sympathetic nerve endings, enhanced β receptor sensitivity, and decreased vagal tone have all been suggested as the underlying cause. Dizziness and confusion have been reported in patients with this syndrome.

Vasovagal syncope

Also referred to as neurogenic, neurovascular or neurocardiogenic syncope, the pathogenesis of the vasovagal attack has been well established. The normal SNS response to a fall in venous return is an increase in sympathetic activity. In vasovagal syncope, a paradoxical fall in SNS activity occurs after a very rapid fall in venous return (Fig. 3.33). The fall in SNS activity may be preceded by a

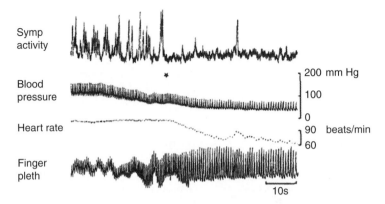

FIGURE 3.33. Changes in muscle sympathetic activity blood pressure, heart rate, and finger pulse plethysmogram during syncope (*asterisk*). (From Wallin BG, Sundlöf G. Sympathetic outflow to muscle during vasovagal syncope. *J Auton Nerv Syst.* 1982;6:287–291.)

short burst of increased sympathetic activity. The lapse in vasoconstrictor activity results in decreased perfusion of the brain, usually preceded by warning signs (ringing in the ears, dizziness) followed by a slow fall to the ground. The supine position is usually followed by prompt recovery.

The cause of the paradoxical sympathetic suppression is unknown but may represent a primitive reflex that evolved in the setting of severe injury where a decrease in SNS activity would be adaptive in terms of decreased energy expenditure and diminished bleeding (hypotension). Increased vagal tone may also occur with slowing of the pulse rate; the latter however is not responsible for the fall in BP, as BP does not respond to atropine.

Shock

Suppression of SNS activity also plays a critical role in the development of shock. Shock may, in some ways, be viewed as a long lasting and severe vasovagal reaction. In experimental studies of shock, prolonged and intense SNS activation is followed by a phase of sympathetic suppression with hypotension. Heart rate may be slowed as well, but is not the cause of the low BP, as vagal blockade with atropine increases heart rate but not BP.

Experimental studies in animals and humans have convincingly demonstrated that hypotension induced by hemorrhage, lower body negative pressure, and acute traumatic injury are associated with SNS suppression. This explains why the administration of adrenergic agonists raises BP in shock, an effect that would not be anticipated in the face of maximally increased endogenous SNS stimulation.

The afferent limb of the reflex decrease in sympathetic activity is not well understood but receptors in the left ventricle appear to be involved.

BIBLIOGRAPHY BY CATEGORY

EXERCISE

Christensen NJ. Sympathetic nervous activity during exercise. *Ann Rev Physiol.* 1983;45: 139–153.

Hartley LH, Mason JW, Hogan RP, et al. Multiple hormonal responses to graded exercise in relation to physical training. *J Appl Physiol.* 1972;33:602–606.

DIETARY INTAKE

Alessi MC, Juhan-Vague I. PAI-1 and the metabolic syndrome. *Arterioscler Thromb Vasc Biol.* 2006;26:2200–2207.

Kaufman LN, Young JB, Landsberg L. Differential catecholamine responses to dietary intake: effects of macronutrients on dopamine and epinephrine excretion in the rat. *Metabolism.* 1989;38:91–99.

Walgren MC, Young JB, Kaufman LN, et al. The effects of various carbohydrates on sympathetic activity in heart and interscapular brown adipose tissue of the rat. *Metabolism.* 1987;36:585–594.

Williams M, Young JB, Rosa RM, et al. Effect of protein ingestion on urinary dopamine excretion. *J Clin Invest.* 1986;78:1687–1693.

Young JB, Landsberg L. Stimulation of the sympathetic nervous system during sucrose feeing. *Nature.* 1977;269:615–617.

Young JB, Landsberg L. Suppression of sympathetic nervous systems during fasting. *Science.* 1977;196:1473–1475.

HYPOGLYCEMIA

Cryer PE. Mechanisms of sympathoadrenal failure and hypoglycemia in diabetes. *J Clin Invest.* 2006;116:1470–1473.

Freinkel N, Metzger BE, Harris E, et al. The hypothermia of hypoglycemia. *N Engl J Med.* 1972;287:841–845.

Orban BO, Routh VH, Levin BE, et al. Direct effects of recurrent hypoglycaemia on adrenal catecholamine release. *Diabet Vasc Dis Res.* 2015;12:2–12.

Rao AD, Bonyhay I, Dankwa J, et al. Baroreflex sensitivity impairment during hypoglycemia— implications for cardiovascular control. *Diabetes.* 2016;65:209–215.

HYPERTENSION

Anderson EA, Hoffman RP, Balon TW, et al. Hyperinsulinemia produces both sympathetic neural activation and vasodilation in normal humans. *J Clin Invest.* 1991;87:2246–2252.

DiBona G. Sympathetic nervous system and hypertension. *Hypertension.* 2013;61:556–560.

Diong C, Jones PP, Tsuchimochi H, et al. Sympathetic hyper-excitation in obesity and pulmonary hypertension: physiological relevance to the 'obesity paradox.' *Int J Obes.* 2016;40:938–946.

Grassi G. Renin-angiotensin-sympathetic crosstalks in hypertension: reappraising the relevance of peripheral interactions. *J Hypertens.* 2001;19:1713–1716.

Grassi G. Counteracting the sympathetic nervous system in essential hypertension. *Curr Opin Nephrol Hypertens.* 2004;13:513–519.

Grassi G. Assessment of sympathetic cardiovascular drive in human hypertension. *Hypertension*. 2009;54:690–697.

Grassi G, Cattaneo BM, Seravalle, et al. Baroreflex control of sympathetic nerve activity in essential and secondary hypertension. *Hypertension*. 1998;31:68–72.

Grassi G, Dell'Oro R, Quarti-Trevano F, et al. Neuroadrenergic and reflex abnormalities in patients with metabolic syndrome. *Diabetologia*. 2005;48:1359–1365.

Grassi G, Seravalle G, Quarti-Trevano F. The 'neuroadrenergic hypothesis' in hypertension: current evidence. *Exp Physiol*. 2010;95(5):581–586.

Joyner MJ, Charkoudian N, Wallin BG. Sympathetic nervous system and blood pressure in humans. *Hypertension*. 2010;56:10–16.

Vollenweider P, Randin D, Tappy L, et al. Impaired insulin-induced sympathetic neural activation and vasodilation in skeletal muscle in obese humans. *J Clin Invest*. 1994;93:2365–2371.

KETOACIDOSIS

Ansstas G, Schade DS, Rubinchik SM et al. Alcoholic Ketoacidosis. Retrieved from http://emedicine.medscape.com/article/116820-overview#showall.

Arky RA, Freinkel N. Alcohol hypoglycemia V. Alcohol infusion to test gluconeogenesis in starvation with special reference to obesity. *N Engl J Med*. 1966;274:426–433.

Devenyi P. Alcoholic hypoglycemia and alcoholic ketoacidosis: sequential events of the same process? *Can Med Assoc J*. 1982;127:513.

Field JB, Williams HE, Mortimore GE. Studies on the mechanism of ethanol-induced hypoglycemia. *J Clin Invest*. 1963;42:497–506.

Foster DW, McGarry JD. The metabolic derangements and treatment of diabetic ketoacidosis. *N Engl J Med*. 1983;309:159–169.

Freinkel N, Arky RA, Singer DL, et al. Alcohol hypoglycemia IV. Current concepts of its pathogenesis. *Diabetes*. 1965;14:350–361.

Fulop M, Ben-Ezra J, Bock J. Alcoholic ketosis. *Alcohol Clin Exp Res*. 1986;10:610–615.

Herrera E, Knopp RH, Freinkel N. Carbohydrate metabolism in pregnancy VI. Plasma fuels, insulin, liver composition, gluconeogenesis, and nitrogen metabolism during late gestation in the fed and fasted rat. *J Clin Invest*. 1969;48:2260–2272.

Mehta A, Emmett M. Fasting ketosis and alcoholic ketoacidosis. In: *UpToDate*. Philadelphia, PA: Wolters Kluwer; 2016.

Miles JM, Haymond MW, Nisse SL, et al. Effects of free fatty acid availability, glucagon excess, and insulin deficiency on ketone body production in postabsorptive man. *J Clin Invest*. 1983;71:1554.

Sinha N, Venkatram S, Diaz-Fuentes G. Starvation ketoacidosis: a cause of severe anion gap metabolic acidosis in pregnancy. *Case Rep Crit Care*. 2014;906283.

Wood ET, Kinlaw WB. Nondiabetic ketoacidosis caused by severe hyperthyroidism. *Thyroid*. 2004;14(8):628–630.

HYPOXIA, HYPERCAPNIA, COPD

Duplain H, Vollenweider L, Delabays A, et al. Augmented sympathetic activation during short-term hypoxia and high-altitude exposure in subjects susceptible to high-altitude pulmonary edema. *Circulation*. 1999;99:1713–1718.

Fletcher EC. Sympathetic over activity in the etiology of hypertension of obstructive sleep apnea. *Sleep*. 2003;1:15–19.

Guyenet PG. Neural structures that mediate sympathoexcitation during hypoxia. *Respir Physiol.* 2000;121:147–162.

Hansen J, Sander M. Sympathetic neural overactivity in healthy humans after prolonged exposure to hypobaric hypoxia. *J Physiol.* 2003;546:921–929.

Heindl S, Lehnert M, Criée CP, et al. Marked sympathetic activation in patients with chronic respiratory failure. *Am J Respir Crit Care Med.* 2001;164:597–601.

Mazzeo RS, Wolfel EE, Butterfield GE, et al. Sympathetic response during 21 days at high altitude (4,300 m) as determined by urinary and arterial catecholamines. *Metabolism.* 1994;43:1226–1232.

Morgan BJ, Crabtree DC, Palta M, et al. Combined hypoxia and hypercapnia evokes long-lasting sympathetic activation in humans. *J Appl Physiol.* 1995;79:205–213.

Rostrup M. Catecholamines, hypoxia and high altitude. *Acta Physiol Scand.* 1998;162:389–399.

Xie A, Skatrud JB, Puleo DS, et al. Exposure to hypoxia produces long-lasting sympathetic activation in humans. *J Appl Physiol.* 2001;91:1555–1562.

SLEEP APNEA

Bratton DJ, Gaisl T, Wons AM, et al. Approaches for lowering blood pressure in patient with obstructive sleep apnea. *JAMA.* 2015;314:2280.

Dopp JM, Reichmuth KJ, Morgan BJ. Obstructive sleep apnea and hypertension: mechanisms, evaluation, and management. *Curr Hypertens Rep* 2007;9:529–534.

Leuenberger UA, Brubaker D, Quraishi SA, et al. Effects of intermittent hypoxia on sympathetic activity and blood pressure in humans. *Auton Neurosci.* 2005;121:87–93.

Somers VK, Mark, AL, Abboud FM. Sympathetic activation by hypoxia and hypercapnia – implications for sleep apnea. *Clin Exp Hypertens A.* 1998;10:413–422.

CONGESTIVE HEART FAILURE

Esler M, Kaye D. Is very high sympathetic tone in heart failure a result of keeping bad company? *Hypertension.* 2003;42:870–872.

Grassi G, Seravalle G, Cattaneo BM, et al. Sympathetic activation and loss of reflex sympathetic control in mild congestive heart failure. *Circulation.* 1995;92:3206–3211.

Hasking GJ, Esler MD, Jennings GL, et al. Norepinephrine spillover to plasma in patients with congestive heart failure: evidence of increased overall and cardiorenal sympathetic nervous activity. *Circulation.* 1986;73:615–621.

Mancia G. Sympathetic activation in congestive heart failure. *Eur Heart J.* 1990;11:3–11.

Triposkiadis F, Karayannis G, Giamouzis G, et al. The sympathetic nervous system in heart failure. *J Am Coll Cardiol.* 2009;54:1747–1762.

THYROID ADRENAL INTERACTION

Landsberg L, Axelrod J. Influence of pituitary, thyroid, and adrenal hormones on norepinephrine turnover and metabolism in the rat heart. *Circ Res.* 1968;22:559–571.

McDevitt DG, Riddell JG, Hadden DR, et al. Catecholamine sensitivity in hyperthyroidism and hypothyroidism. *Br J Clin Pharm.* 1978;6:297–301.

Ribeiro MO, Carvalho SD, Schultz JJ, et al. Thyroid hormone-sympathetic interaction and adaptive thermogenesis are thyroid hormone receptor isoform-specific. *J Clin Invest.* 2001;108:97–105.

SYNCOPE AND SHOCK

The Consensus Committee of the American Autonomic Society and the American Academy of Neurology. Consensus statement of the definition of orthostatic hypotension, pure autonomic failure, and multiple system atrophy. *Neurology.* 1996;46:1470.

Dietz NM, Joyner MJ, Shepherd JT. Vasovagal syncope and skeletal muscle vasodilation: the continuing conundrum. *Pacing Clin Electrophysiol.* 1997;20:775–780.

Freeman R. Neurogenic orthostatic hypotension. *N Engl J Med.* 2008;358:615–624.

Öberg B, Thorén P. Circulatory Responses to Stimulation of Left Ventricular Receptors in the Cat. *Acta Physiol Scand.* 1973;88:8–22.

Pålsson J, Ricksten SE, Delle M, et al. Changes in renal sympathetic nerve activity during experimental septic and endotoxin shock in conscious rats. *Circ Shock.* 1988;24:133–141.

Rea RF, Wallin BG. Sympathetic nerve activity in arm and leg muscles during lower body negative pressure in humans. *J Appl Physiol.* 1989;66:2778–2781.

Ryan KL, Rickards CA, Hinojosa-Laborde C, et al. Sympathetic responses to central hypovolemia: new insights from microneurographic recordings. *Front Physiol.* 2012;3:1–14.

Schadt JC, Ludbrook J. Hemodynamic and neurohumoral responses to acute hypovolemia in conscious mammals. *Am J Physiol.* 1991;260:H305–H318.

Wallin BG, Sundlöf G. Sympathetic outflow to muscles during vasovagal syncope. *J Auton Nerv Syst.* 1982;6:287–291.

Young JB, Fish S, Landsberg L. Sympathetic nervous system and adrenal medullary responses to ischemic injury in mice. *Am J Physiol.* 1983;245:E67–E73.

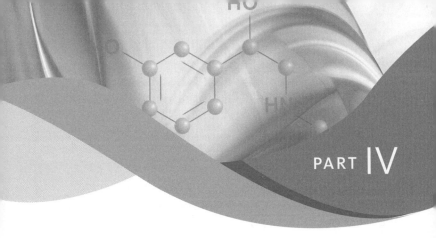

PART IV

Pharmacology

Drugs that affect adrenergic functions are among the most commonly employed therapeutic agents in medical practice. The adrenergic pharmaceuticals that constitute the therapeutic armamentarium may affect adrenergic receptors, sympathetic nerve endings, or central sympathetic outflow. Most of these agents are congeners of the naturally occurring catecholamines.

Adrenergic Agonists

Adrenergic agonists are compounds that stimulate adrenergic receptors and produce the characteristic response of the stimulated effector tissue. Adrenergic receptors are considered in detail in Part I.

Therapeutic uses of the naturally occurring catecholamines

Although not extensively used anymore because of their nonselective effects, brief duration of action, and requirement for parenteral administration, the naturally occurring catecholamines do have important therapeutic indications and are lifesaving in some situations (Table 4.1).

Epinephrine

The most important use of E is in the treatment of severe allergic reactions, particularly anaphylaxis, where the prompt administration of E is frequently lifesaving. Patients with bee venom allergy or idiopathic anaphylaxis should be instructed in the use of Epi Pens for immediate subcutaneous or intramuscular self-administration upon exposure or at the beginning of an attack. When patients present in shock from anaphylaxis, intravenous (i.v.) E should be administered

TABLE 4.1	Therapeutic Uses of the Naturally Occurring Catecholamines

Epinephrine
Anaphylaxis
   Insect venom
   Idiopathic anaphylaxis
   Severe hypersensitivity reactions (facial swelling, bronchospasm)
Cardiac arrest
   Intravenous or intracardiac
Combination with local anesthetics (prolong duration of action, delay absorption)

Norepinephrine
Hypotension, shock

Dopamine (dose-dependent effects)
Hypotension
   Low dose: ↑ renal, mesenteric blood flow (DA1 receptors)
   Higher dose: ↑ cardiac stimulation (β_1 receptors)
   Highest dose: ↑ vasoconstriction, ↑ BP (α_1 receptors)

DA, dopamine; BP, blood pressure.

through a secure i.v. line. It is essential to use the proper dilution as E comes in vials of different strengths. When given by the i.v. route, it should be diluted and administered slowly. The usual dose by this route is about 0.3 to 0.5 mg; the dose can be titrated to the restoration of blood pressure (BP) in patients with severe hypotension. E is the specific antidote for anaphylactic reactions; diphenhydramine (Benadryl) and other antihistamines have a secondary role.

E is also used as a cardiac stimulant in cardiac arrests; it may be administered i.v. or *via* intracardiac injection. Other uses include combination with topical anesthetic agents to delay absorption and prolong the effect, and as a topically applied agent to decrease bleeding.

Norepinephrine

NE, a potent pressor, is used in the treatment of shock and severe hypotensive reactions. It should be administered through an indwelling i.v. line to avoid extravasation with subsequent necrosis and sloughing of the skin.

Dopamine

Intravenous DA has a range of effects that depend on the concentration achieved in the blood; at low rates of infusion, stimulation of the DA1 receptors results in renal and mesenteric vasodilation and increased sodium excretion, actions that are beneficial in some clinical situations associated with low BP and poor renal perfusion. At higher rates of infusion, it stimulates β_1 receptors and exerts a positive inotropic and chronotropic effect on the heart. At further higher concentrations, α_1 receptors are stimulated with an increase in vasoconstriction and hence BP. Some of the effects of DA are exerted indirectly by releasing NE from SNS terminals. These actions make DA a potentially useful agent in the treatment of hypotensive oliguric states such as congestive heart failure (CHF), hepatorenal syndrome, and shock.

Sympathomimetic amines

Congeners of the naturally occurring catecholamines that stimulate adrenergic receptors are referred to as sympathomimetic amines because they mimic, in some respects, the actions of endogenous catecholamines or the effects of SNS stimulation (Tables 4.2 and 4.3). The basic parent compound is phenylethyl-amine with the carbon atoms designated as shown in Figure 1.1. The structure–activity relationships for sympathomimetic amines have been well established: substitutions and deletions at various sites account for the different patterns of activity, receptor subtype selectivity, oral bioavailability, differences in metabolism,

TABLE 4.2	Direct Acting Sympathomimetic Amines		
Agonist	Receptor	Effect	Common indication
Phenylephrine (i.v.)	α_1	Vasoconstriction	Hypotension; PAT
Midodrine (oral)	α_1	Vasoconstriction	Orthostatic hypotension; Hepatorenal syndrome
Clonidine (oral; dermal patch)	α_2 (CNS)	SNS suppression	Hypertension
α-Methyldopa (oral)	α (CNS)	SNS suppression	Hypertension in pregnancy
Isoproterenol (i.v.)	β_1, β_2	Cardiac stimulation; Bronchodilation	Bradycardias; Torsade de pointes
Albuterol (inhaler)	β_2	Bronchodilation	Asthma (rescue inhaler)
Terbutaline (oral; s.c.; inhaler)	β_2	Bronchodilation	Asthma (acute attack)
Formoterol (long-acting inhaler)	β_2	Bronchodilation	Asthma (chronic treatment)
Salmeterol (long-acting inhaler)	β_2	Bronchodilation	Asthma (chronic treatment)
Dobutamine (i.v.)	$\beta_1, \beta_2, \alpha_1$	↑ Cardiac contractility	CHF
Pseudoephedrine (oral)	$\alpha_1, \alpha_2, \beta_2$	Vasoconstriction; bronchodilation	Decongestant (allergies, URIs)

i.v., intravenous; s.c., subcutaneous; CNS, central nervous system; SNS, sympathetic nervous system; PAT, paroxysmal atrial tachycardia; CHF, congestive heart failure; URI, upper respiratory infection.

TABLE 4.3	Indirect and Mixed Acting Sympathomimetic Amines		
Agonist	Receptor	Effect	Common indication
Ephedrine (oral) (direct + indirect)	α, β	CV and CNS stimulation; Bronchodilation	Rarely prescribed
Amphetamine (oral) (indirect)	α, β	CNS and CV stimulation; Appetite suppressant	Rarely prescribed; ADHD; narcolepsy; obesity
Methylphenidate (oral) (Indirect)	α, β	CNS stimulation	ADHD; narcolepsy

CV, cardiovascular; CNS, central nervous system; ADHD, attention deficit/hyperactivity disorder.

prolongation of action, and for central nervous system (CNS) penetration, as compared with the naturally occurring catecholamines and with each other. A few salient points about the synthetic molecular modifications include the following: (1) metabolism is altered and the duration of action prolonged by modifications of the catechol structure (blocks metabolism by catechol O-methyltransferase) and by substitutions on the α carbon of the side chain (blocks metabolism by monoamine oxidase [MAO]); (2) absence of a polar (hydroxyl) group on the β carbon of the side chain increases lipid solubility and CNS penetration; and (3) substitution of alkyl groups for hydrogen on the amino nitrogen conveys β receptor (particularly β_2) activity.

Direct and indirect acting sympathomimetic amines

Sympathomimetic amines may also be classified as direct or indirect acting: the direct acting compounds stimulate adrenergic receptors, whereas the indirect acting amines release NE from the neurotransmitter stores in the sympathetic nerve endings. Indirect acting sympathomimetic amines are substrates for the amine uptake process of the SNS endings; once they gain access to the nerve ending, they may release NE from storage sites in the granules of the nerve terminals, thereby generating a sympathomimetic effect. These indirect acting amines may also block NE reuptake into the nerve ending, thus potentiating the adrenergic response. Tyramine is the prototypical indirect acting amine, whereas phenylephrine is the prototypical direct acting α_1 agonist. Many sympathomimetic amines exhibit both direct and indirect effects. Because they release NE, indirect acting sympathomimetic amines have both α and β effects.

Some indirect acting amines may be stored in the sympathetic granules and released in response to sympathetic nerve impulses. As these amines are less potent than the endogenous neurotransmitter NE, the subsequent effector response is diminished. These compounds are referred to as "false transmitters."

α Adrenergic agonists

Many sympathetic amines have been developed with substantial selectivity for the α or β receptor as well as for the various subtypes of both groups. The second messengers and intracellular cascades in effector tissues are considered in Part I.

Selective α₁ receptor agonists and their therapeutic applications

Phenylephrine causes smooth muscle contraction including, most importantly, vasoconstriction; it is used as a nasal decongestant, for pupillary dilatation, and as a vasopressor. Although there is an oral formulation that has been marketed as an alternative to pseudoephedrine, its effectiveness by the oral route has been questioned; its major use as a decongestant for colds and allergies is as a nasal spray. It is particularly useful as an i.v. pressor agent for hypotension induced by spinal anesthesia, and may be useful for the treatment of hypotension associated with sepsis as well. In patients with paroxysmal atrial tachycardia, it has been used to elevate BP as a means of sharply increasing vagal tone in order to convert back to sinus rhythm.

Oxymetazoline is an imidazoline derivative utilized as a locally applied direct acting α_1 agonist that causes vasoconstriction; it is used as a decongestant in nasal sprays for symptomatic relief of allergies, upper respiratory infections, and sinus congestion. In topical ophthalmic preparations, it is used for allergic conjunctivitis. Other imidazoline derivatives are also available for similar topical usage.

Midodrine, a prodrug that forms the active metabolite desglymidodrine, is a selective α_1 agonist that causes vasoconstriction of the arterial and venous vascular beds. It is active after oral ingestion and has a duration of action of 4 to 6 hours. It is used in the treatment of orthostatic hypotension but its efficacy is limited by supine hypertension and venoconstriction, which diminishes the reservoir in the capacitance vessels, an effect that may worsen the orthostatic fall in BP. It is frequently employed in cirrhotic patients with low BP, oliguria, and impending hepatorenal syndrome, again with limited efficacy.

Droxidopa (L-dihydroxyphenylserine, L-DOPS), although not a selective α_1 inhibitor, is another prodrug used in the treatment of orthostatic hypotension. A synthetic amino acid precursor of NE, droxidopa is decarboxylated by L-aromatic amino acid decarboxylase to form NE in vivo. The NE so formed functions as a circulating vasopressor rather than as a neurotransmitter. It is administered orally and has a duration of action of about 4 to 6 hours. It increases BP in the sitting and standing positions without an increase in heart rate. The supine position must be avoided to prevent severe hypertension (black box warning). Use of this drug requires supervision and it is not established that efficacy is retained after long-term usage. Like all treatment for neurogenic orthostatic hypotension, it is less than satisfactory as it does not restore the normal relationship between changes in position and SNS activity. It may, nonetheless, provide symptomatic improvement in some patients.

Selective α_2 receptor agonists and their therapeutic applications

Clonidine, a centrally acting α_2 agonist, diminishes central sympathetic outflow via an inhibitory effect on brainstem sympathetic centers, thereby lowering BP. Its major use is in the treatment of hypertension. It is active orally and also available as a transdermal patch that releases active compound over a period of 1 week. Clonidine has been used in the treatment of addictions where it may ameliorate withdrawal symptoms in patients addicted to narcotics, alcohol, and benzodiazepines. The usefulness of clonidine is limited by a host of adverse effects, many reflective of its actions on the CNS. These include drowsiness, fatigue, dry mouth, vivid dreams and nightmares, and hallucinations. Abrupt withdrawal of clonidine may result in reflexive SNS discharge with a hypertensive paroxysm, so discontinuation of clonidine should be gradual rather than abrupt.

α-**Methyldopa** is a prodrug that is decarboxylated to α-methyldopamine and β-hydroxylated to α-methylnorepinephrine. It acts in the brainstem as a false neurotransmitter to stimulate α_2 receptors, which in turn restrain SNS outflow. High concentrations may develop in the brain as it is not a substrate for MAO. Once widely used in the treatment of hypertension, immunologic reactions such as a positive Coombs test and occasionally hemolytic anemia, as well as sedation and hepatotoxicity have precluded its general usefulness; however, it is still utilized in the treatment of hypertension in pregnancy as it is effective and safe for both fetus and mother.

β Receptor agonists

Isoproterenol is the prototypic, synthetic, nonselective β agonist. It relaxes vascular and visceral smooth muscle resulting in decreased peripheral resistance and bronchodilation. It stimulates the heart increasing cardiac contractility and heart rate, thereby increasing cardiac output and myocardial oxygen consumption. It has very limited therapeutic application, reserved principally for increasing the heart rate in patients with bradycardia or heart block pending pacemaker placement. It may also be used in the treatment of *torsade de pointes* to increase heart rate and shorten the QT interval. The development of selective β_2 agonists has replaced nonspecific β agonists like isoproterenol, E, and ephedrine in the treatment of bronchospasm.

Selective β_2 receptor agonists

Selective β_2 agonists were developed to capture β receptor–mediated bronchodi-lation without the cardiac stimulation that is the prominent response engendered by nonselective β agonists. The selectivity of β_2 agonists is however only relative; at high doses, β_1-mediated cardiac stimulation does occur.

Short-acting β_2 agonists are used predominantly by inhalation to abort acute attacks of wheezing in asthmatic patients ("rescue inhalers"). **Albuterol** is the most commonly used β_2 agonist. It is available as an oral preparation but most commonly prescribed for inhalation. The effect is rapid in onset (about

15 minutes) and the duration of action is about 3 to 4 hours. Major side effects include tachycardia (β_1 stimulation) and tremulousness. **Terbutaline** is another short-acting β_2 agonist available for treating bronchospasm; it is available for oral administration and for subcutaneous injection as well as by inhalation. Its off-label use as a tocolytic agent to produce uterine relaxation in the treatment of preterm labor is no longer recommended because of serious maternal and fetal side effects.

Long-acting β_2 agonists are used as inhalation bronchodilators in the treatment of asthma and chronic obstructive pulmonary disease. **Formoterol** and **salmeterol** are long-acting, lipophilic, highly selective β_2 agonists. They have a duration of action of over 12 hours making them suitable for the treatment of chronic obstructive pulmonary disease (COPD) and nocturnal asthma. They are usually given in combination with inhaled corticosteroids or anticholinergics. Formoterol has a rapid onset of action in comparison with salmeterol.

Sympathomimetic amines with mixed actions

Dobutamine, a congener of DA that was originally developed as a selective agonist of the β_1 receptor, is now recognized to have a much more complex mechanism of action. It stimulates β_1, β_2, and α_1 adrenergic receptors resulting in a positive inotropic effect with little increase in heart rate and with little or no increase in BP. It is administered as an i.v. infusion and is useful for the short-term treatment of CHF.

Ephedrine is both a direct and indirect acting sympathomimetic amine. It stimulates α and β receptors directly and releases NE from the sympathetic nerve endings. In times past, it was used in the treatment of asthma, heart block, and to promote weight loss, but has been replaced by newer more selective agents. It causes an increase in BP and CNS stimulation, especially in association with large doses. Although it is no longer prescribed, it is an important and unquantified constituent of herbal concoctions such as ma huang and *Ephedra*, available in health food stores and in alternative medicine outlets, and confers considerable risk when taken unsupervised in large amounts.

Pseudoephedrine acts directly on α and β_2 receptors causing vasoconstriction and bronchodilation. It is used as an oral decongestant in allergic rhinitis and upper respiratory infections. It is effective and safe and sold over the counter often in combination with antihistamines; its sale, however, is restricted because it can easily be converted to methamphetamine in "home" laboratories.

Amphetamine is an orally active indirect acting sympathomimetic amine with strong stimulatory CNS effects. It also stimulates the cardiovascular system resulting in significant BP elevation. The *d*-isomer (dextroampetamine, dexedrine) has more powerful CNS effects than the racemic compound. The central alerting effects are due to release of NE from central neurons with a lesser contribution from the release of DA. It suppresses appetite and has been used off-label as an adjunct for weight loss, but safety considerations and potential for abuse preclude its usage for weight reduction. It is FDA approved for narcolepsy and attention deficit/hyperactivity disorder (ADHD), but is not commonly used for these indications.

Methamphetamine is a centrally active congener of amphetamine that releases NE and DA at central synapses and potentiates central catecholamine action by blocking reuptake and inhibiting MAO. It is a major drug of abuse and has no therapeutic uses.

Methylphenidate (Ritalin), another congener of amphetamine, with a similar mechanism of action is commonly used in the treatment of ADHD and occasionally for narcolepsy. It helps ADHD patients concentrate and improves school performance. It is a controlled substance and its use should be carefully supervised. It is contraindicated in glaucoma.

Phentermine is an orally active congener of amphetamine that suppresses appetite and is used, frequently in combination with other agents, in the treatment of obesity.

Adrenergic Antagonists

Many widely used therapeutic agents antagonize the effects of sympathoadrenal stimulation. These agents have a high degree of selectivity for α or β adrenergic receptors as well as for a number of subtypes of each of the classic receptors. As a consequence of the wide range of pharmacologic activity of adrenergic receptor antagonists, a number of highly useful applications have been developed and these encompass many therapeutic indications.

α Receptor antagonists

Nonselective α receptor antagonists block the full range of responses at both α_1 and α_2 receptors. The development of selective α_1-blockers has greatly diminished the usefulness of the older nonselective α antagonists. **Phentolamine** produces a short-acting competitive blockade of both α_1 and α_2 receptors. It is usually administered intravenously. Its major use is in the treatment of hypertensive paroxysms in patients with pheochromocytoma. It may also be injected locally to prevent necrosis in areas of the skin where accidental extravasation of NE has occurred during i.v. infusion. Side effects are related to α receptor antagonism, notably hypotension. Nonselective α antagonists block the presynaptic inhibition (α_2-mediated) of NE release; the resulting increase in NE spillover in the synaptic cleft stimulates the cardiac β receptors resulting in tachycardia; this does not occur with α_1 selective agents as α_2-mediated suppression of NE release remains intact.

Phenoxybenzamine (dibenzyline) produces a long-acting irreversible noncompetitive blockade of α receptors. These properties make phenoxybenzamine an ideal agent for the treatment of patients with pheochromocytoma, which is the only current indication for its use. It is given orally, twice daily, titrating the dose up slowly to normalize the BP and avoid, insofar as possible, orthostatic hypotension. In patients with pheochromocytoma, α blockade antagonizes arterial and venous constriction, lowers BP and expands plasma volume, and improves carbohydrate metabolism by increasing insulin secretion, the latter by blocking the suppressive effect of catecholamines (α-mediated) on insulin release.

Selective α_1 antagonists

Although cloning has identified several subtypes of the α_1 receptor (designated 1a–d), the clinical relevance of the different subtypes is questionable in the absence of subtype-specific agonists and antagonists (Table 4.4). All the selective α_1-blockers affect vascular smooth muscle on both arteries and veins as well as urinary bladder trigone, sphincter, and prostate gland smooth muscle. The prominent effect is to relax vascular smooth muscle resulting in hypotension without an increase in heart rate, in distinction to the tachycardia that accompanies nonselective α blockade. Both preload and afterload are reduced because of the effect on both arteries and veins.

Prazosin, terazosin, doxazosin, and tamsulosin

Prazosin was the first α_1 selective agent in general clinical use but suffered from a short half-life and a duration of action of just 7 to 10 hours, necessitating inconvenient dosing intervals. **Terazosin** has a longer duration of action than prazosin but still less than 24 hours. **Doxazosin** has a much longer half-life, is suitable for once a day dosing, and as a consequence is the most commonly used agent of the three. Terazosin and doxazosin are used to treat hypertension and lower urinary tract symptoms related to benign prostatic hypertrophy (BPH).

TABLE 4.4	α Receptor Antagonists
Phentolamine (i.v.) Short-acting, competitive blockade	Pressor crises in pheochromocytoma; MAOI interactions, clonidine withdrawal, cocaine overdose
Phenoxybenzamine (oral) Long-acting noncompetitive blockade	Pheochromocytoma
Selective α_1-blockers Prazosin (oral) Short-acting competitive blockade	Pressor crises
Terazosin (oral) Intermediate acting competitive blockade	Hypertension, BPH
Doxazosin (oral) Long-acting competitive blockade	Hypertension, BPH
Tamsulosin (oral) Intermediate acting competitive blockade	BPH

i.v., intravenous; MAOI, monoamine oxidase inhibitor; BPH, benign prostatic hypertrophy.

These agents have a favorable side effect profile and improve insulin sensitivity and glucose metabolism, but are not first-line antihypertensive agents because the possibility that doxazosin precipitated CHF was raised in the ALLHAT trial. Their use in BPH continues but has been surpassed by another α_1 selective agent **tamsulosin**, which has some selectivity for the prostate and causes less hypotension. All of these agents can cause orthostatic hypotension, particularly with the initial dose; they are generally given at night before bed. Their usefulness in BPH depends upon antagonism of spasm of the urinary bladder and trigone.

Doxazosin has proven efficacy in the preoperative treatment of pheochromocytoma particularly when phenoxybenzamine is not available. Prazosin is useful for the treatment of hypertensive paroxysms in patients with pheochromocytoma as control is being established with the longer acting agents, and in the treatment of pressor crises that occur with MAO inhibitors, cocaine-induced hypertension, or with clonidine withdrawal.

β Receptor antagonists ("β-blockers")

β receptor antagonists are among the most commonly prescribed drugs. They have a wide application, principally in the therapy of cardiovascular disease, but also in noncardiac diseases (Table 4.5). A bewildering array of β-blockers have been developed and a variety of pharmacologic effects have been noted in different compounds, some of which convey useful activities in addition to β blockade, some of which alter the pharmacokinetics, and some of which have no obvious clinical significance. Three main groups of β-blockers may be distinguished on the basis of their major pharmacologic characteristics (Table 4.6): nonselective β-blockers (so-called first generation); β_1 selective blockers (cardioselective, second generation); and vasodilating β-blockers (third generation). Other

TABLE 4.5	Indications and Contraindications for β Blockade
Indications for β-blockers	**Contraindications for β-blockers**
Ischemic heart disease	Asthma, COPD
Acute MI	Cardiac conduction abnormalities
Post MI	Cocaine-induced hypertensive crisis
Angina pectoris	Cocaine-induced MI
Congestive heart failure	Raynaud's phenomena
Dissecting aortic aneurysm	Obesity, metabolic syndrome
Marfan's syndrome	Insulin resistance
Hypertension	Hyperkalemia
Hyperthyroidism	
Pheochromocytoma (after α blockade)	
Portal hypertension	
Essential tremor	
Migraine prophylaxis	

MI, myocardial infarction; COPD, chronic obstructive pulmonary disease.

TABLE 4.6	First, Second, and Third Generation β-Blockers

Nonselective β-blockers (first generation)
Propranolol (oral, blocks β_1 and β_2 receptors)
    Therapeutic uses: hyperthyroidism; pheochromocytoma (after α blockade);
        portal hypertension; tachycardias; migraine prophylaxis; essential tremor
Nadolol (long duration of action)

Cardioselective β_1-blockers (second generation)
Metoprolol (oral, i.v.)
    Therapeutic uses: MI; post MI; angina; hypertension; CHF; tachycardia
Atenolol (oral, long duration of action)
    Therapeutic uses: hypertension; hyperthyroidism; hypertrophic cardiomyopathy
Esmolol (i.v., short duration of action)
    Used in ORs and ICUs for tachycardia and aortic dissection

Vasodilating β-blockers (third generation)
Carvedilol (oral, blocks β_1, β_2, α_1 receptors)
    Therapeutic uses: CHF; hypertension; MI
Labetolol (oral, i.v., blocks β_1, β_2, α_1 receptors)
    Therapeutic uses: Hypertensive crises (ER, OR, ICU)

i.v., intravenous; MI, myocardial infarction; CHF, congestive heart failure; OR, operating room; ICU, intensive care unit; ER, emergency room.

properties such as lipid solubility, membrane stabilization, and local anesthetic effects influence CNS penetration, volume of distribution, and duration of action. Some β-blockers have intrinsic agonist activity for the receptor; as partial agonists, they may cause less of a fall in resting heart rate but are very rarely used. Membrane stabilizing effects do not contribute to the antiarrhythmic efficacy of β blockade; all the major pharmacologic effects depend upon antagonizing activation of the β receptor.

A major increase in functionality for the β-blockers was achieved by adding the capacity for vasodilation to the β blockade. Vasodilation depends on different mechanisms in the various third generation blockers, including nitric acid production, β_2 agonism, α_1 blockade, and calcium channel blockade. Concomitant vasodilation reduces afterload (useful in the treatment of CHF) and diminishes insulin resistance (improving glucose metabolism and the lipid profile).

Indications for β blockade

Ischemic heart disease remains a major indication for the use of β blockade, a predictable consequence of the known effects of these agents on the heart. Heart rate, contractile state, and wall tension are the major determinants of myocardial oxygen consumption; all of these are increased by catecholamines and antagonized by β blockade. These well-established effects have made β blockade a cornerstone in the symptomatic treatment of angina pectoris, although it should be noted that these agents have not been demonstrated to decrease the likelihood of subsequent events in patients with stable coronary artery disease. The efficacy of β blockade in diminishing mortality in patients with **acute myocardial infarction** (absent a significant contraindication) and **postmyocardial infarction** is also well established.

CHF is another widely accepted indication for β blockade. After the introduction of β blocking agents, CHF was considered a significant contraindication to their use, and caution is still required as the negative inotropic effects may initially worsen CHF, but long-term efficacy of β blockade in the treatment of CHF has been demonstrated and is now widely accepted. Slowing the heart rate and decreasing myocardial oxygen consumption are presumably involved in the beneficial effect.

Dissecting aortic aneurysm, particularly those involving the descending thoracic aorta, constitutes another indication for β blockade as the propagation of the clot in the false lumen depends upon the rate of ventricular contraction (dP/dt), a physiologic variable antagonized by β-blockers. β blockade is a crucial part of the antihypertensive regimen in the treatment of aortic dissection. In patients with **Marfan's syndrome,** β blockade may be of prophylactic benefit in reducing the rate of aortic dilatation and perhaps diminishing the likelihood of dissection, although this latter point is controversial.

Hypertension was, in times past, a disease frequently treated with β blocking agents. The antihypertensive effect of β blockade is still incompletely understood, but is multifactorial, including a decrease in cardiac output, suppression of renin release, and perhaps an inhibition of central SNS outflow. Currently, β-blockers are not considered first-line antihypertensive drugs for the following reasons: they may increase peripheral resistance; they have adverse metabolic effects on insulin resistance which includes an increase in the likelihood of developing type 2 diabetes as well as an increase in triglycerides and a decrease in high-density lipoprotein (HDL)-cholesterol; they are associated with (modest) weight gain. These adverse factors are significantly mitigated in third generation vasodilating β-blockers. For the present β blockade should not be used as first-line agents in the therapy of hypertension absent a specific indication such as ischemic heart disease.

Thyrotoxicosis is a well-established indication for β blockade. Nonselective agents (propranolol, atenolol) are preferred. The major beneficial effects are to counteract the sympathomimetic features of thyroid hormone excess. Thus, palpitations, tachycardia, tremor, anxiety, widened palpebral fissure (stare), and rapid reflex return are all ameliorated. Heat intolerance may be improved but effects on metabolic rate are minimal. At high dosage, propranolol inhibits the peripheral conversion of triiodothyronine to thyroxine but this is not a major effect at the usual doses employed.

Pheochromocytoma is an important indication for the use of β-blockers, with the crucial proviso that they not be administered until after α adrenergic blockade is initiated, in order to prevent unopposed α receptor stimulation. In patients with pheochromocytoma, β blockade has the following beneficial effects: ↓tachycardia, palpitations; ↓metabolic rate, sweating; and, critically important, antagonizing anesthesia-induced arrhythmias.

Portal hypertension is another indication for nonselective β blockade which diminishes portal pressure and protects against recurrent variceal hemorrhage.

Essential tremor, migraine prophylaxis, and **open-angle glaucoma** (ophthalmic drops) are additional indications for β-blockers.

Contraindications (or precautions) in the use of β blockade

Asthma and **COPD** are important, although not absolute, contraindications to the use of β-blockers. Sporadic mild bronchospasm does not preclude use of selective β_1 agents, although careful observation is required under these circumstances (Table 4.5).

Cardiac conduction abnormalities constitute an important, and frequently overlooked, contraindication to β blockade. First-degree atrioventricular block and bilateral bundle branch block (QRS duration longer than 0.12, bifascicular block) are harbingers of complete heart block which may be precipitated by β-blockers as these drugs slow intraventricular conduction.

Cocaine-induced hypertensive crisis, the result of neuronal uptake blockade with consequent amplification of sympathetic discharge, is a contraindication to β blockade as it accentuates the hypertension by rendering α receptor stimulation unopposed. This is true for **cocaine-induced myocardial infarction** as well.

Raynaud's phenomenon may be worsened by β blockade as the latter is associated with a decrease in cardiac output and an increase in peripheral resistance.

Obesity and the **metabolic syndrome** constitute relative contraindications to the use of β-blockers, as these agents are associated with weight gain, insulin resistance, a characteristic dyslipidemia (low HDL-cholesterol, high triglycerides), and an increased propensity to develop type 2 diabetes. β-blockers may, however, be used in the presence of obesity and the metabolic syndrome for a compelling cardiac indication such as myocardial infarction.

Hyperkalemia may be accentuated by β blockade which antagonizes catecholamine mediated potassium uptake into cells. This necessitates careful monitoring of β blocking agents in patients on spironolactone or other potassium-sparing diuretics as well as angiotensin blockers and angiotensin-converting enzyme inhibitors.

Nonselective (first generation) β-blockers

Propranolol is the prototypic β adrenergic blocker. It blocks β_1 and β_2 receptors (Table 4.6). Although newer agents with β_1 selectivity and other properties such as vasodilation have replaced propranolol for a number of indications, propranolol still is considered first line in the treatment of thyrotoxicosis, in the treatment of pheochromocytoma, and in the prophylaxis of variceal hemorrhage in patients with cirrhosis and portal hypertension. **Nadolol** is another nonselective β-blocker with a much longer half-life; it is used much less frequently than propranolol.

Cardioselective (second generation) β_1-blockers

The three most commonly used β_1 selective blockers are **metoprolol, atenolol, and esmolol**, each of which has indications that favor its usage. It should be noted that β_1 selectivity is only relative and far less than the selectivity afforded by α_1 agents as compared with nonselective α-blockers. **Metoprolol** is usually favored by cardiologists for ischemic heart disease; it has a short duration of action so is usually given twice per day, but a delayed release form is available for once a day dosing. **Atenolol** has a long duration of action and is frequently used in the treatment of hypertension and hyperthyroidism. β_1 selective agents are also very useful in patients with hypertrophic cardiomyopathy and in those with diastolic dysfunction; for these indications, angiotensin II inhibitors and calcium channel blockers are frequently used as well in combination or singly. **Esmolol** has a very brief duration of action and is used intravenously in situations where rapid onset and offset are desirable, such as in the operating room or the intensive care unit. It is useful in slowing the heart rate in situations where tachycardia threatens the circulation, and in the treatment of tachyarrhythmias including supraventricular tachycardias.

Vasodilating (third generation) β-blockers

The third generation vasodilating β-blockers are increasingly used in the treatment of hypertension and CHF. The two most commonly used agents are **labetalol** and **carvedilol**; both of these agents block β_1, β_2, and α_1 adrenergic receptors. The clinical usage of these two drugs is, however, very different. **Labetalol** is available as an oral and i.v. preparation and approved for the treatment of hypertension but its major use is via the i.v. route for the treatment of acute severe hypertensive crises. It is principally used in the emergency room, the operating theater, and the intensive care unit. It has a complex pharmacology because it exists as a mixture of racemic forms. The potency of blockade of the β receptor is much greater than the blocking effect on the α receptor by a factor of 5 to 10 times. It has a rapid onset of action by the i.v. route and a duration of action of a few hours. **Carvedilol** has its principal use as an oral agent in the treatment of hypertension and CHF. The vasodilating properties lessen the adverse impact that β blockade has on insulin resistance and carbohydrate and lipid metabolism.

Other third generation β-blockers include **bucindolol**, **celiprolol**, and **betaxolol**.

Drugs Affecting the Metabolism and the Inactivation of Catecholamines

Monoamine oxidase inhibition

MAO inhibition is a widely distributed mitochondrial flavoprotein that oxidatively deaminates amines with the production of the corresponding aldehyde and ammonia. The aldehyde is subsequently oxidized to the corresponding acid or reduced to the corresponding glycol. There are two isoforms of the enzyme designated MAO A and MAO B based on substrate specificity and tissue localization. Neurons contain both forms; MAO A is present in virtually all mammalian cells (save erythrocytes), whereas MAO B outside the nervous system is limited to platelets. MAO functions to metabolize circulating amines, principally in the gut, the liver, and the kidney. It plays an important role in catecholamine metabolism but not, as discussed in Part I, in the termination of action at the adrenergic receptors. Within the peripheral adrenergic nerve endings, MAO regulates the neuronal stores of NE by deaminating cytoplasmic NE; when MAO is inhibited, the neuronal concentration of NE is significantly increased.

Monoamine oxidase inhibitors (MAOI) are utilized in the treatment of severe depression and, specifically MAO B inhibitors, in the treatment of Parkinson's disease. Agents that inhibit MAO A are associated with reactions that affect the peripheral SNS, namely predisposition to **pressor crises** and the formation of **false neurotransmitters**. Both these reactions depend upon tyramine (4-hydroxyphenylethylamine), an indirect acting sympathomimetic amine, which is formed in foods from the decarboxylation of the amino acid tyrosine. As the latter reaction results from the action of bacterial decarboxylases during fermentation reactions, the concentration of tyramine in particular foodstuffs is hard to predict with accuracy, but commonly noted rich sources include meat extracts and pickled herring, red wines, beers and ales, fava beans, sauerkraut, and chocolate. When MAO is inhibited, dietary tyramine escapes deamination in the gut and the liver and gains access to the circulation where it is taken up by the sympathetic nerve endings. When ingested in large quantities, tyramine releases NE from the enhanced stores in the SNS producing the typical **pressor crisis**. The latter resembles the pressor crises seen with pheochromocytoma and cocaine overdose: headache, palpitations, sweating, and markedly increased BP. Other indirect acting sympathomimetic amines, such as those that occur in nonprescription cold or allergy medications, also produce the pressor reactions, and therefore should be avoided in patients taking MAOI. Treatment is with a short-acting α-blocker; β-blockers are to be avoided under these circumstances.

Paradoxically, MAOI are also associated with hypotension, particularly orthostatic hypotension. Small amounts of tyramine, gradually taken up by the SNS when MAO is inhibited, accumulate in the storage vesicles and are β-hydroxylated to octopamine, which dilutes the NE storage pool. Octopamine is released along with NE in response to sympathetic impulses (**false neurotransmitter**) and because it is a weaker vasopressor than NE, a reduced sympathetic response is the result.

Cocaine
Cocaine blocks the neuronal uptake of NE; as reuptake is the major inactivation mechanism at adrenergic synapses, blockade of NE reuptake by cocaine is associated with potentiated SNS responses. Central sympathetic activity is increased

as well. In response to a cocaine overdose, accentuated SNS activity results in a typical **pressor crisis** with tachycardia, palpitations, sweating, and extreme BP elevations. Cocaine-induced myocardial infarction is a well-recognized complication and may result from increases in myocardial oxygen consumption and in some cases coronary artery vasospasm. Cardiac arrhythmias may also occur and, rarely, aortic dissection has been noted. Skeletal muscle vasoconstriction with rhabdomyolysis and myoglobinuric renal failure is also a well-known complication of cocaine overdose. Enhanced SNS responses underlie all these complications of cocaine overdose.

BIBLIOGRAPHY BY CATEGORY

GENERAL
Westfall TC, Westfall DP. Adrenergic agonists and antagonists. In: Brunton LL, Chabner BA, Knollmann BC, eds. *Goodman & Gilman's The Pharmacological Basis of Therapeutics.* 12th ed. New York, NY: McGraw-Hill; 2011.

α BLOCKADE & BPH
Lepor H. Alpha blockers for the treatment of benign prostatic hyperplasia. *Rev Urol.* 2007;4:181–190.

COCAINE
Schwartz BG, Rezkalla S, Kloner RA. Cardiovascular effects of cocaine. *Circulation.* 2010;122:2558–2569.

MAO INHIBITORS
Holschneider DP, Shih JC. Monoamine oxidase: basic and clinical perspectives. Brentwood, TN: American College of Neuropsychopharmacology; 2000.

Youdim MBH, Edmondson D, Tipton KF. The therapeutic potential of monoamine oxidase inhibitors. *Neuroscience.* 2006;7:295–309.

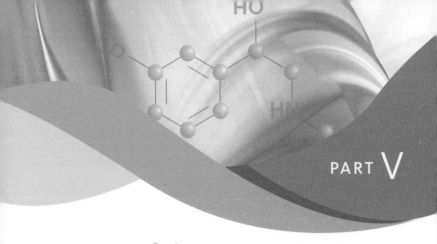

PART V

Tumors of the
Sympathoadrenal System

Tumors of the sympathoadrenal system include pheochromocytomas, paragangliomas, ganglioneuromas, ganglioneuroblastomas (GNBs), and neuroblastomas (NBs). These tumors arise from primitive sympathoadrenal cell precursors in the neural crest (Fig. 5.1) which differentiate into mature adrenal chromaffin cells, extra-adrenal chromaffin cells, and sympathetic ganglion cells. At each stage of maturation, transformation into tumors may occur as shown in Figure 5.1.

Pheochromocytoma

The chromaffin cell

Pheochromocytoma, by far the most clinically important of the group of sympathoadrenal tumors, arise from chromaffin cells, principally in the adrenal medulla, but also in extra-adrenal locations. The portmanteau term chromaffin implies an affinity for chromium salts, derived from the fact that the cut surface of the adrenal medulla darkens markedly on exposure to potassium dichromate; the dichromate oxidizes the catecholamines which polymerize to highly pigmented compounds that turn the tissue black (Fig. 5.2) when applied to the cut surface of the tumor. Formerly used in confirming the diagnosis, it has been replaced by identifying neuroendocrine markers and by the characteristic electron photomicrograph appearance which clearly demonstrates chromaffin granules. Extra-adrenal pheochromocytomas are also called paragangliomas (Fig. 5.1). Some tumors arising from parasympathetic ganglia, particularly in

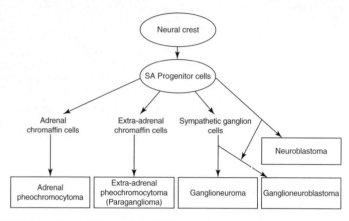

FIGURE 5.1. Genesis of tumors derived from the sympathoadrenal system.

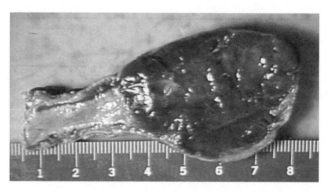

FIGURE 5.2. The gross appearance of pheochromocytoma ranges from *pink-tan* to *yellow* to *slightly brown*. The freshly cut tumor surface turns *dark brown* **(right half of image)** when immersed in potassium dichromate solution (pH between 5 and 6). This is caused by oxidation of stored catecholamines synthesized by the tumor and is known as the chromaffin reaction. (From the University of Alabama at Birmingham Department of Pathology PEIR Digital Library© [http://peir.net].)

the head and neck, do not secrete catecholamines but are also referred to as paragangliomas. The term "pheo" is just a shortened, convenient designation for pheochromocytoma.

Incidence and importance

Pheochromocytoma is an uncommon disease: it has been estimated that between 0.1% and 0.2% of the hypertensive population harbors a pheochromocytoma. Even so, given the prevalence of hypertension, the incidence of undiagnosed patients with pheochromocytoma is not insignificant. In fact, unselected autopsy series indicate that a great majority of pheochromocytomas are not diagnosed during life, even though the tumor is responsible for the death in most of these cases. The relative rarity of pheochromocytoma, therefore, should not obscure its importance: promptly diagnosed and properly treated pheochromocytoma is usually completely curable; if the diagnosis is missed, or if the disease is improperly treated, death is the usual outcome.

The clinical manifestations of pheochromocytoma are due to the unregulated release of catecholamines from the tumor. As a consequence, alarming and occasionally catastrophic signs and symptoms can occur, obscuring the diagnosis, and confounding proper management. In some cases, other biologically active compounds may be released, producing distinctive clinical manifestations (Table 5.1).

Pheochromocytoma is usually solitary and sporadic but a significant minority of patients have pheochromocytoma as part of an inherited syndrome. In these cases, bilateral, multiple, and extra-adrenal tumors frequently occur.

Location

In adults, about 80% of pheochromocytomas are sporadic, solitary, nonmalignant tumors located in or about a single adrenal, 10% are bilateral, 10% are extra-adrenal, and about 10% are malignant. In children, bilateral and extra-adrenal pheos are more common than in adults. Bilateral adrenal pheochromocytomas always indicate an inherited syndrome and necessitate genetic screening. Extra-adrenal pheos are located in or about the sympathetic ganglia and reflect the embryonic location of extra-adrenal chromaffin cells (Fig. 5.3). Most occur within the abdomen around the preaortic plexuses including the celiac, the superior mesenteric, and the inferior mesenteric ganglia. About 10% of the extra-adrenal pheos occur in the thorax usually around the paraspinal sympathetic ganglia. One percent are located in the urinary bladder. Approximately 3% may be found in the head

TABLE 5.1	Peptide Hormones Produced and Secreted by Pheochromocytomas
Hormone	**Clinical association**[a]
Adrenomedullin	Hypotension, shock
ACTH	Ectopic ACTH syndrome (Cushing's syndrome)
VIP	Watery diarrhea, hypokalemia, achlorhydria (WDHA) syndrome
PTHrP	Hypercalcemia
Erythropoietin	Polycythemia
Interleukin-6	Fever, systemic inflammatory response syndrome

ACTH, adrenocorticotropic hormone; VIP, vasoactive intestinal peptide; PTHrP, parathyroid hormone-related protein.
[a] See text for details.

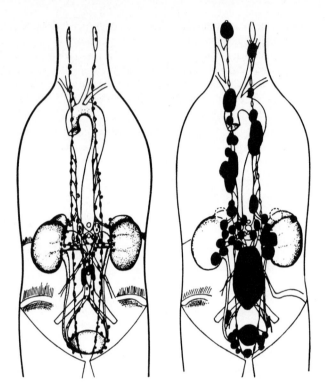

FIGURE 5.3. Distribution of chromaffin tissue in the newborn compared with the distribution of extra-adrenal pheochromocytomas. Extra-adrenal pheochromocytomas **(right)** occur in sites containing chromaffin tissue in the newborn **(left)**. (From Landsberg L, Young JB. *Williams Textbook of Endocrinology*. Philadelphia, PA: WB Saunders; 1992:621–705.)

and neck either with the sympathetic ganglia or the extracranial branches of the 9th or 10th cranial nerves, although these rarely secrete catecholamines. Isolated case reports indicate that pheochromocytomas may occur in a variety of other locations within viscera.

Pathology

Pheochromocytomas are very vascular. As such, they are subject to hemorrhage and necrosis, as seen on the cut surface of these tumors (Figs. 5.2 and 5.4). Necrosis in the tumor leads to release of stored catecholamines resulting in the paroxysm that characterizes pheochromocytoma; the surgical specimen frequently shows a fresh hemorrhage, presumably responsible for the hypertensive crisis that brought the patient to medical attention.

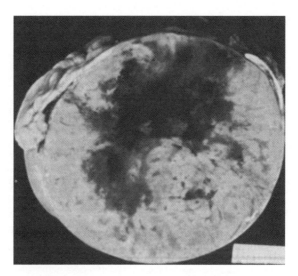

FIGURE 5.4.   Adrenal pheochromocytoma showing cut surface. The marker is 1 cm. Note the normal adrenal surrounding the tumor, and extensive hemorrhage and necrosis. (From Landsberg L, Young JB. *Williams Textbook of Endocrinology*. Philadelphia, PA: WB Saunders, 1992:621–705.)

Most adrenal pheochromocytomas weigh less than 100 g and are less than 10 cm in diameter, but very large tumors, softball size, occasionally occur. Extra-adrenal pheos are typically smaller weighing between 20 and 40 g and measuring less than 5 cm in diameter.

Microscopically, pheos consist of large pleomorphic chromaffin cells containing chromaffin granules strikingly demonstrated by electron microscopy. They stain positive for chromogranin A and other markers indicative of a neural origin such as synaptophysin and tyrosine hydroxylase. Malignancy occurs in less than 10% of pheos overall; extra-adrenal pheos that are part of genetic paraganglioma (PGL) syndromes are more likely to be malignant. Malignancy cannot be determined by the histologic features or even by local invasion; distant metastases are the only sure measure of malignancy but a variety of features suggesting aggressiveness have been described such as high cellularity, confluent necrosis, vascular invasion, aneuploidy or tetraploidy, and an increase in mitotic figures. Metastases, when these occur, are found in lymph nodes, bone, liver, and lung.

Catecholamine storage and release

The synthesis and storage of catecholamines in pheochromocytomas resemble those same processes that occur in the normal adrenal medulla. The mechanisms of release of these compounds from the tumor, however, are poorly understood because pheochromocytomas, unlike the normal adrenal medulla, are not innervated. It seems likely that necrosis, changes in blood flow, and external pressure may be involved in triggering release. A number of drugs used therapeutically and diagnostically have the capacity to stimulate release from the tumor, occasionally with catastrophic results, as described below.

Adrenal pheos produce both NE and E, with the percentage of NE generally exceeding that found in the normal adrenal medulla. This is reflected in the urinary catecholamine excretion pattern: NE is most commonly the predominant catecholamine excreted. An important exception is in the multiple endocrine neoplasia type 2 (MEN 2) syndromes described below. In these cases, E predominates and early on elevated urinary E is the only abnormality. Extra-adrenal pheochromocytomas secrete NE exclusively with the vanishingly rare exception of extra-adrenal tumors that contain phenylethanolamine-n-methyltransferase (PNMT) and produce E as well as NE. The predominant catecholamine secreted cannot be predicted from the constellation of symptoms. Increased secretion of dopamine (DA) or its major metabolite homovanillic acid (HVA) is much more common in malignant than the usual benign tumor, although increased DA exertion is not diagnostic of malignancy.

Other bioactive compounds released from pheochromocytomas

Pheos produce and secrete a variety of hormones and mediators that may contribute to the clinical presentation (Table 5.1). Most notable and clinically relevant are corticotropin (adrenocorticotropic hormone—ACTH), adrenomedullin, parathyroid hormone-related protein (PTHrP), vasoactive intestinal peptide (VIP), erythropoietin, and interleukin-6 (IL-6).

Typical clinical features

The clinical manifestations of pheochromocytoma reflect the unrestrained release of catecholamines and other bioactive substances from the tumor.

The paroxysm is the defining feature of pheochromocytoma (Table 5.2). Episodic headache, sweating, and palpitations constitute the classic symptom triad. The typical pressor crisis or paroxysm occurs as a presenting manifestation in about half the patients with pheochromocytoma. If the blood pressure is taken during one of these episodes, it will almost always be elevated, often to alarming levels. The opportunity to observe and record the BP during a symptomatic episode has, therefore, significant diagnostic importance.

Paroxysms last from minutes to hours and occur at variable intervals, although as the disease progresses, they tend to occur more frequently and to be more severe. In addition to the classic triad of headache, palpitation, and sweating, chest or abdominal pain with nausea and vomiting are common. Pallor or flushing may be associated. The abdominal pain may be severe and frequently reflects hemorrhage within the tumor; hemorrhagic necrosis is frequently responsible for the catecholamine release that causes the crisis.

Although the paroxysm is the most distinctive feature of pheo, **hypertension** is the most common clinical manifestation, occurring in almost all cases that are

TABLE 5.2	**The Typical Paroxysm**
Episodic, unregulated release of catecholamines	

Symptoms and signs:
  Headache, sweating and palpitations
  Very high BP (frequently with tachycardia)
  Chest or abdominal pain
  Pallor/flush
  Apprehension (sense of impending doom)	

Duration: 5 min to an hour (or longer)	
Frequency: Episodic; variable periodicity (more frequent and severe over time)	

BP, blood pressure.

diagnosed clinically. The hypertension is sustained in about 60% of patients with pheochromocytoma; in the remainder, it is episodic, occurring mostly during paroxysms (Table 5.3).

As about half the patients with a pheo do not have discreet spells or paroxysms, it is useful to consider when pheo should be suspected in hypertensive patients (Table 5.4). This is important because pheo patients with sustained high blood pressure and no paroxysms masquerade as essential hypertension. There are, however, clues that suggest the need to rule out pheochromocytoma in hypertensive patients. These include: hypertension of new onset; young age; very high BP; malignant hypertension defined by fibrinoid necrosis of arterioles manifesting clinically as flame hemorrhages in the eye grounds, retinal infarctions (cotton wool spots), and heavy proteinuria and/or hematuria; incidental adrenal mass on imaging; recent weight loss; tachycardia; high hematocrit; marked BP lability; new carbohydrate intolerance; and when orthostatic hypotension is present in the untreated state. As pheochromocytoma is a rare disease, it will need to be excluded much more often than ruled in. The consequences of missing the diagnosis, as noted above, are grave.

TABLE 5.3	**Hypertension in Pheochromocytoma**

Sustained 60%
  With crises 27%
  Without crises 33%	

Paroxysmal 30% Normotensive between attacks	
No hypertension 10% Discovered incidentally or through screening	

TABLE 5.4	Features in Hypertensive Patients That Warrant Screening for Pheochromocytoma
Spells of any kind	
Weight loss	
Recent onset of hypertension	
Young age	
Severe or malignant hypertension	
Tachycardia	
Marked BP lability	
Carbohydrate intolerance or overt new onset diabetes mellitus	
Adrenal mass on imaging	
Orthostatic hypotension in untreated state	
Family history of pheo	
Unanticipated prominent changes in BP (up or down) in response to drugs or diagnostic manipulations	

BP, blood pressure.

Other distinctive clinical features and underlying pathophysiology

The **orthostatic hypotension**, frequently noted in patients with pheo, is due principally to venoconstriction and diminished plasma volume (Table 5.5). The body cannot assess volume status directly but is very good at measuring changes in pressure; the surrogate measure for volume, pressure in the capacitance portion of the circulation (great veins) is, therefore, the afferent signal for changes in volume. Under ordinary circumstances, an increase in pressure in the great vein signifies volume expansion ("a full tank") and initiates a diuresis to maintain extracellular fluid balance. Catecholamine-stimulated venoconstriction in patients with a pheo increases pressure in the venous system, thereby simulating volume expansion and initiating a diuresis which results in decreased plasma volume. Rather than a "full tank," patients with a pheo have a smaller tank. The decreased plasma volume impairs the normal physiologic response to upright posture, which entails maintaining venous return by shifting blood from the capacitance vessels to the heart thus maintaining cardiac output.

An additional contributing factor to the orthostatic fall in BP may be the loss of reflex tone in the SNS because of the high circulating catecholamine levels.

Carbohydrate intolerance is common in patients with pheo and overt diabetes mellitus is not rare; the major factor responsible is suppression of insulin by the direct effect of catecholamines on the pancreatic beta cells. Alpha adrenergic blockade will release the restraint on insulin and restore carbohydrate metabolism toward normal in most cases. Surgical removal frequently reverses the impairment in carbohydrate resulting in a "cure" of the diabetes.

Increased metabolic rate in pheochromocytoma patients is another common pathophysiologic manifestation. The stimulation of thermogenesis results in sweating, not fever, as the temperature set point is not altered. Weight loss is

TABLE 5.5	**Some Other Manifestations of Pheochromocytoma**
Carbohydrate intolerance   Suppression of insulin; glycogenolysis and gluconeogenesis

Increased metabolic rate
  Stimulation of nonshivering thermogenesis (BAT)
    Weight loss; sweating

Increased hematocrit
  Decreased plasma volume ("stress polycythemia")
  Erythrocytosis (erythropoietin production)

Rhabdomyolysis
  Intense vasoconstriction → muscle necrosis
  Myoglobinuric renal failure

Ischemic colitis
Cardiac ischemia   Increased oxygen demand; coronary artery spasm
Congestive heart failure   Hypertension, myocardial fibrosis
Cholelithiasis
Shock with multiorgan failure and ARDS (shock lung)   Adrenomedullin release
Fever with SIRS   IL-6 production

BAT, brown adipose tissue; ARDS, acute respiratory distress syndrome; SIRS, systemic inflammatory response syndrome; IL, interleukin.

common in pheo patients because of the increased thermogenesis. The old adage "forget a fat pheo" is based on this propensity toward weight loss; pheo does occur in obese patients but generally they will have lost weight prior to initial presentation. **Fever** occurs in a small minority of patients because of the production of IL-6 by the tumor.

Cardiac manifestations are also common in pheo patients. **Cardiac ischemia**, manifested by typical angina due to increased myocardial oxygen demand ($\uparrow$ BP, $\uparrow$contractile state, $\uparrow$wall tension) and/or transmural infarction secondary to coronary artery spasm have been noted. Coronary spasm is inferred from normal coronary arteries at angiography in the face of a transmural infarct. **Congestive heart failure** secondary to hypertension, cardiac hypertrophy, and catecholamine-induced **myocardial fibrosis** also occurs. A variety of arrhythmias and conduction disturbances have also been noted.

A **high hematocrit** may be present, reflecting either reduced plasma volume ("stress" polycythemia from venoconstriction) or, less commonly, actual erythrocytosis from ectopic erythropoietin production. **Hypercalcemia** may also occur due to the production of PTHrP. The incidence of **cholelithiasis** is increased as well in pheochromocytoma patients. Intense vasoconstriction may cause muscle necrosis (**rhabdomyolysis**) or **ischemic colitis**.

Rarely, IL-6 production by the pheo results in an acute and sometimes recurrent, **systemic inflammatory response syndrome.** Associated symptoms include fever, chills, headache, shortness of breath, leukocytosis, and increased levels of inflammatory markers.

Presentation of pheochromocytoma

Pheochromocytoma may present in a variety of ways that suggest other diseases, thereby obscuring the correct diagnosis (Table 5.6). The two most common presentations are hypertension and spells (paroxysms) suggesting essential hypertension on the one hand and panic attacks or epilepsy on the other. Another common presenting manifestation is an unusual blood pressure response (either up or down) to therapeutic or diagnostic interventions. It is said that one out of 20,000 general anesthesias uncovers an unsuspected pheo. Fentanyl, in particular, widely used as a preanesthetic medication, has been well documented to induce a paroxysm, and occasionally these have been fatal. Other less common modes of presentation include: an adrenal mass on imaging for some other indication (adrenal incidentaloma); severe hypotension with noncardiogenic pulmonary edema (shock lung); an abdominal catastrophe with pain and shock (hemorrhage into the tumor); and screening of asymptomatic persons within a kindred of syndromic pheochromocytoma (described in subsequent sections).

Based on autopsy series of consecutive cases of pheochromocytoma from the Mayo Clinic, the majority of cases of pheochromocytoma were not suspected clinically and many were asymptomatic or manifested only nonspecific symptoms.

Adrenal "incidentalomas"

Adrenal incidentalomas are lesions of 1 cm or more discovered incidentally on imaging the abdomen. The prevalence is about 4% on average as judged from

TABLE 5.6	The Many Presentations of Pheochromocytoma
Hypertension	
Spells (seizures, panic attacks)	
Unusual hypertensive or hypotensive response to therapeutic or diagnostic interventions	
Noncardiogenic pulmonary edema (shock lung, ARDS)	
Abdominal catastrophe (hemorrhage into tumor, shock)	
Systemic inflammatory response syndrome with intermittent fever	
Adrenal mass on unrelated imaging	
Screening (families with syndromic pheos in the pedigree)	
Unsuspected during life (found at postmortem examination)	

ARDS, acute respiratory distress syndrome.

autopsy and computed tomography (CT) studies; they occur more commonly in the elderly. About 5% of adrenal incidentalomas turn out to be pheochromocytomas. Although phenotypic appearance on imaging may suggest that pheo is more or less likely, expert consensus favors ruling out pheochromocytoma in all incidentaloma patients before diagnostic tests, such as fine needle aspiration, are performed. This is best achieved by measuring fractionated catecholamines and metanephrines in a 24-hour urine specimen, as described below.

Adverse drug interactions

Adverse drug reactions are responsible for significant morbidity and mortality in patients with pheochromocytoma; in many instances, these reactions trigger a life-threatening paroxysm that leads to the diagnosis (Table 5.7). The adverse drug reactions in pheo patients are of three major types: direct release of catecholamines from the tumor; impairment in catecholamine inactivation; and release of catecholamines from augmented tissue stores in sympathetic nerve endings. Of these, by far the most significant and the most dangerous are the agents that directly release catecholamines from the tumor. Of the latter group, **opioids** are the most important and arguably among the least appreciated offenders.

In an unfortunate, but not rare scenario, patients with an unsuspected pheochromocytoma presenting to an emergency room with headache and high blood pressure receive an opiate for pain relief; the blood pressure increases and the pain worsens, resulting in an additional opiate dose which leads to further worsening and sometimes death. As pheos may also present with chest or abdominal pain, opiate administration may lead to disastrous results in these situations as well.

TABLE 5.7	Adverse Drug Reactions in Patients with Pheochromocytoma
Release of catecholamines from the tumor	
Opioids	
Metoclopramide	
Glucagon	
Histamine	
Glucocorticoids	
ACTH	
Intra-arterial radiographic contrast media	
Blockade of neuronal uptake of catecholamines	
Tricyclic antidepressants	
Cocaine	
Inhibition of metabolism of catecholamines	
MAO inhibitors	
Indirect acting sympathomimetic amines	
Nasal decongestants	

ACTH, adrenocorticotropic hormone; MAO, monoamine oxidase.

Tachycardia and very high blood pressure, sometimes with wide swings, should raise the possibility of a pheo. Fentanyl, administered as a preanesthetic, may also cause a pressor crisis as noted above.

Other agents that directly release catecholamines from the tumor include metoclopramide, glucagon, histamine, glucocorticoids, and ACTH. Radiographic contrast media, when delivered intra-arterially to the tumor is well recognized to produce pressor crises, but intravenous (i.v.) administration is perfectly safe.

Agents that interfere with the metabolic disposition of catecholamines also increase BP and worsen symptoms in patients with pheochromocytoma. Antidepressants that block the neuronal uptake of catecholamines, notably tricyclics, are the major offenders. These agents do not provoke pressor crises but accentuate the effects of catecholamines on blood pressure. Monoamine oxidase (MAO) inhibitors increase the store of catecholamines in the sympathetic nerve endings, thereby accentuating SNS responses.

The third class of agents that worsen BP in patients with pheochromocytoma are indirect acting sympathomimetic amines. These drugs, most of which are available over the counter as nasal decongestants, release the augmented stores of catecholamines in the SNS, thereby increasing blood pressure.

In patents with known pheochromocytoma, the administration of all drugs should be carefully considered.

Syndromic pheochromocytoma

Somewhere in the neighborhood of 25% to 30% of pheos are inherited, most commonly as part of distinct familial syndromes, including MEN 2A and B, retinal cerebellar hemangioblastomatosis (von Hippel–Lindau disease, VHL), neurofibromatosis type 1 (NF1), PGL syndromes type 1 and 4 (succinic dehydrogenase subtype D—SDHD and subtype B—SDHB), and several other less common genetic mutations (Table 5.8). All of the above reflect germline mutations and are inherited as autosomal dominant traits. Heritable pheos tend to occur at earlier ages than the more common sporadic variety (less than 45 years old). Bilateral and/or multiple pheos are virtually always inherited. Genetic screens are available for all the common mutations associated with syndromic pheos. For NF1, however, clinical criteria usually suffice to establish the presence of the trait and recourse to genetic screening is rarely done for NF1.

MEN Syndromes

The **MEN 2** syndrome is caused by a mutation in the RET protooncogene which codes for a transmembrane tyrosine kinase; the mutation results in constitutive activation of the tyrosine kinase which induces tumor formation in the affected endocrine glands. In MEN 2A, the mutation is in the extracellular domain of the RET protein, whereas in MEN 2B, the intracellular domain is affected.

MEN 2A (Sipple's syndrome) is a triad consisting of medullary carcinoma of the thyroid (MTC), pheochromocytoma, and hyperparathyroidism. Virtually all

TABLE 5.8	Syndromic Pheochromocytoma		
Syndrome	Mutation	Pheochromocytoma	Associated diseases
MEN 2A	RET →↑ TK	Bilateral adrenal	MTC; hyperpara
MEN 2B	RET →↑ TK	Bilateral adrenal	MTC; mucosal neuromas
VHL	↑HIF→↑ VEGF	Bilateral adrenal; extra-adrenal	Hemangioblastomas; renal cell carcinoma
NF1	↑ RAS	Bilateral adrenal	Neurofibromas; Café au lait spots; skeletal abnormalities
PGL 1	SDHD → ↑ HIF → ↑ VEGF	Extra-adrenal; bilateral adrenal	—
PGL 4	SDHB → ↑ HIF → ↑ VEGF	Extra-adrenal; bilateral adrenal, ↑ malignancy	—

See text for details.

MEN, multiple endocrine neoplasia; VHL, von Hippel–Lindau disease; NF, neurofibromatosis; PGL, paraganglioma; RET, ???; TK, tyrosine kinase; HIF, hypoxia-inducible factor; VEGF, vascular endothelial growth factor; RAS, ???; SDHD, succinic dehydrogenase subtype D; SDHB, succinic dehydrogenase subtype B; MTC, medullary carcinoma of the thyroid.

affected individuals either have or will develop MTC which begins as parafollicular C cell hyperplasia and necessitates thyroidectomy in all cases. About 50% of affected individuals have or will develop a pheochromocytoma which has unique characteristics as described below. Less than 25% have or will develop hyperparathyroidism which may be in the form of single or multiple adenomas or hyperplasia.

MEN 2B (mucosal neuroma syndrome) consists of MTC, pheochromocytoma, and mucosal neuromas involving the eyelids and the lips giving a characteristic appearance (Fig. 5.5) of glistening bumps. Intestinal ganglioneuromas and Marfanoid habitus are occasionally prominent. Although the mucosal neuromas are apparent from childhood, the diagnosis is frequently delayed until late adolescence or early adulthood when symptoms of a pheo or a neck mass bring the patient to medical attention. The MTC occurs earlier and is more aggressive as compared with the MEN 2A syndrome. In distinction to the MEN 2A, a family history in MEN 2B is frequently absent, suggesting that a *de novo* mutation may be more common in this syndrome. The characteristics of the pheos are similar in the MEN 2A and 2B syndromes.

The pheochromocytomas in the MEN syndromes begin as adrenal medullary hyperplasia which leads to multicentric intra-adrenal lesions (Fig. 5.6). E secretion is prominent and early in the evolution of these lesions, elevated E excretion is the only abnormality. This has important implications in screening family members in MEN kindreds: it is necessary to measure E in a 24-hour urine collection.

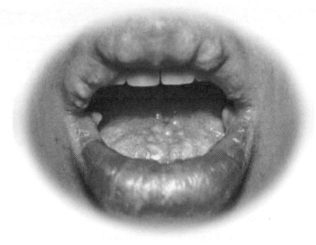

FIGURE 5.5. Mucosal neuromas.

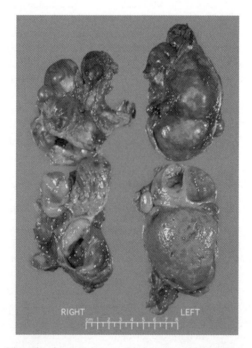

FIGURE 5.6. Bilateral multicentric lesions with discrete nodules are shown. (From AFIP Atlas of Tumor Pathology.)

Extra-adrenal pheos (paragangliomas) do not occur in the MEN syndromes and the incidence of malignant pheochromocytoma is vanishingly rare. In both MEN 2 syndromes, the clinical presentation of a pheo in the propositus has frequently served to identify an affected kindred.

Although all patients with the MEN 2 syndrome require total thyroidectomy once the RET genetic mutation is established, pheochromocytoma must be excluded or removed prior to thyroid surgery.

von Hippel–Lindau retinal cerebellar hemangioblastomatosis

The VHL gene encodes a tumor suppressor protein that increases the activity of a hypoxia-inducible factor (HIF) which in turn activates vascular endothelial growth factor (VEGF) and other potential tumorigenic compounds. Many different germline mutations have been described in kindreds with the VHL syndrome. The VHL syndrome includes pheochromocytoma, hemangioblastomas of the nervous system and retina, renal cell carcinoma, and neuroendocrine tumors of the pancreas.

The occurrence of pheochromocytoma in the VHL syndrome is highly variable in different kindreds with a VHL germline mutation; depending on the particular mutation, pheo may be absent or present in a high percentage of patients. Within a particular kindred, the presence of a pheochromocytoma indicates that all affected subjects in that kindred are at risk of the development of a pheo. The characteristics of pheochromocytomas in the VHL syndrome include a high incidence of bilateral adrenal lesions and the occasional presence of extra-adrenal pheos (paragangliomas) principally in the abdomen but also in the thorax. Malignant pheos occur, but rarely.

Neurofibromatosis type 1

The product of the NF1 gene blocks the inactivation of the oncogene RAS. Between 1 and 2% of patients with NF1 (also known as von Recklinghausen's disease) develop pheochromocytomas although the percentage is higher in NF1 patients with hypertension and in NF1 patients in postmortem series. Stigmata of neurofibromatosis are usually present, including multiple café au lait spots, characteristic neurofibromas, and skeletal abnormalities particularly involving the spine. The pheochromocytomas may be bilateral, and extra-adrenal pheos do occur, although they are not particularly common. Malignancy occurs in about 10%, similar to the rate in sporadic pheos.

Paraganglioma syndromes

Germline mutations in the enzyme succinic acid dehydrogenase (SDH) are responsible for the familial PGL syndromes. This enzyme, which functions as a component both of the Kreb's cycle and the mitochondrial electron transport chain, consists of four subunits; mutations in each of the subunits, designated A, B, C, and D, produce different phenotypes. The molecular pathogenesis involves HIF, as does the VHL mutation. HIF degradation is impaired in these syndromes inducing a pseudo-hypoxic state which increases VEGF and other mitogenic factors leading to tumor formation. The germline mutation produces susceptibility to tumor formation; somatic inactivation of the normal allele leads to tumor development. The hypoxic theory is buttressed by the reported increase in paragangliomas in children with cyanotic congenital heart disease.

The important mutations causing pheochromocytomas and paragangliomas involve the D (PGL 1) and B (PGL 4) subunits of SDH. **PGL 1** is associated with a high incidence of bilateral adrenal pheochromocytomas and paraganglioma. The pheos are not malignant. **PGL 4** also has a high incidence of bilateral adrenal pheos and paragangliomas but malignancy is more common than in sporadic pheos, or in the other syndromic pheos.

Pheochromocytoma of the urinary bladder

Pheochromocytoma may, very rarely, occur in any viscera but location in the urinary bladder has attracted particular attention because of the association of paroxysms with micturition, a manifestation obviously caused by contraction of the detrusor muscle with release of catecholamines from the tumor. About 50% of patients have pressor crises during urination with headache, hypertension, and palpitation being the most common symptoms. Other symptoms include palpitations, sweating, and occasional syncope. Hematuria occurs in about half the patients. Of particular importance is the fact that a significant minority of patients have normal catecholamine measurements, presumably because these tumors become symptomatic at an earlier stage of their development. These tumors can be seen by modern imaging techniques and at cystoscopy.

Diagnosis of pheochromocytoma

The trick in diagnosing pheochromocytoma is to think of it. As it is a rare disease and the manifestations are not specific, the possibility of pheochromocytoma may not be considered in the initial differential diagnosis. Knowledge of the various presentations outlined above may help bring this diagnosis to mind.

The diagnosis is established by the demonstration of increased catecholamine production (Table 5.9). This is usually accomplished by measuring free (unconjugated) fractionated catecholamines (NE, E, DA) and metanephrines (normetanephrine [NMN], metanephrine [MN]) in a 24-hour urine collection. Alternatively, plasma-free metanephrines may be used either initially for screening or for conformation. Much has been written about the various tests in terms of sensitivity and specificity; the Endocrine Society practice guidelines favor plasma metanephrines, whereas the Mayo Clinic recommends 24-hour urine for catecholamines and metanephrines as the initial screening test in most circumstances. If there is any doubt, measurements for both urinary catecholamines and metanephrines and plasma metanephrines should be obtained. Twenty-four–hour urine specimens should be measured for creatinine as well to insure the adequacy of collection.

In most patients with pheochromocytoma, substantial elevations (at least three times the normal upper limit) of catecholamines and metanephrines will establish

TABLE 5.9	**Laboratory Tests for Pheochromocytoma**
24-hour urine collection (upper limits[a])	
Free (unconjugated) fractionated catecholamines:	
NE 170 μg/24 h; E 35μg/24 h; DA 700 μg/24 h	
Free (unconjugated) fractionated metanephrines:	
NMN 900 μg/24 h; MN 400 μg/24 h	
Plasma	
Free (unconjugated) fractionated metanephrines:	
NMN 0.66 nmol/L; MN 0.3 nmol/L	

Determinations by high-pressure liquid chromatography with electrochemical detection.

E, epinephrine; DA, dopamine; MN, metanephrine; NE, norepinephrine; NMN, normetanephrine.

[a] Values may vary in different laboratories

the diagnosis. Minor elevations just outside the upper limits very rarely turn out to be pheos. Pheos in the urinary bladder are an exception to this venerable rule.

The great majority of patients with pheochromocytoma will be diagnosed with the first properly performed assay for catecholamines and metanephrines. Normal values make the diagnosis extremely unlikely. The problem is that pheo is a difficult diagnosis to exclude with absolute certainty, especially in patients with persistent symptoms, because small tumors and those that secrete intermittently may (rarely) have normal values. In patients with spells or paroxysmal hypertension, normal values may rarely be obtained in the interictal periods, although most patients with intermittent symptoms will have elevated catecholamines and metanephrines all the time, even when they are asymptomatic. In evaluating patients with spells, a 24-hour urine collection should be initiated right after the attack begins and continued for the next 24 hours. Normal values for catecholamines and metanephrines make pheo very unlikely as a cause of the spells.

Current assays are performed by high-pressure liquid chromatography (HPLC) with electrochemical detection or mass spectroscopy. These assays, to a large extent, eliminate the problem of interfering substances that plagued the older fluorescent assays but a number of drugs still may elevate the measured levels of catecholamines and metanephrines. These include some β blockers, MAO inhibitors, L-DOPA and α-methyl DOPA, tricyclic antidepressants, cocaine, and phenoxybenzamine among others. Clinicians should confer with the clinical laboratory performing the assay about interfering substances and to ascertain the appropriate precautions relating to sample acquisition.

Modern assays have rendered the older pharmacologic provocative (glucagon, histamine) and blocking (phentolamine) tests obsolete; safety considerations appropriately preclude their use.

Differential diagnosis

Pheochromocytoma is a rare disease with clinical features that resemble, sometimes closely, other more common entities (Table 5.10). Most of these can rather easily

TABLE 5.10	**Differential Diagnosis**	
	NE/NMN	Diagnosis
Hyperthyroidism	Normal	↑T4, ↑T3, ↓TSH
Carcinoid syndrome	Normal	↑5-HIAA urinary
Hyperadrenergic essential hypertension	Normal	Negative imaging
Pressor crises		
Cocaine	+/− ↑	Drug screen/history
MAOI + tyramine	↑NMN	History
Clonidine withdrawal	+/− ↑	History
Intracranial catastrophe	↑	Imaging/coma
Factitious	+/− ↑	Psych history

MAOI, monoamine oxidase inhibitors; NE, norepinephrine; NMN, normetanephrine; TSH, thyroid stimulating hormone; 5-HIAA, 5-hydroxy indole acetic acid.

be excluded by a careful consideration of the clinical features; in others, a properly performed analysis for catecholamines and metanephrines in a 24-hour urine collection, as described above, will be required to rule out pheochromocytoma.

Hyperthyroidism, for example, superficially resembles pheo because of weight loss, sweating, palpitations, and tremor. Although the systolic BP may be increased in hyperthyroidism, the diastolic BP is usually low; the wide pulse pressure reflects the increase in cardiac output that occurs in hyperthyroidism. Thyroid function tests easily establish the correct diagnosis.

The **carcinoid syndrome**, because of episodic flushing along with the mistaken belief that carcinoid is associated with hypertension, may also be confused with pheochromocytoma. The carcinoid syndrome, however, is associated with kinin-induced hypotension, not hypertension, and the characteristic flush is in distinction to the pallor usually associated with pressor crises in patients with a pheo. Elevated urinary 5-hydroxy-indole acetic acid, the major metabolite of serotonin, establishes the diagnosis.

The most significant problem lies in differentiating pheochromocytoma from essential hypertension with hyperadrenergic features, the so-called **pseudopheochromocytoma**. These patients, who may have sweating and tachycardia, and occasional palpitations, suffer from an overactive SNS. Measurements of catecholamines and catecholamine metabolites are usually normal, but may be borderline elevated, thereby causing confusion and leading to an extensive search for a small extra-adrenal pheo. These patients virtually never turn out to have a pheo. Imaging studies, described below, may be helpful in ending the futile search for the nonexistent tumor.

Pressor crises caused by drugs or drug withdrawal may transiently increase catecholamine excretion but can readily be excluded by history. Major offenders include cocaine, clonidine withdrawal, MAO inhibitors plus tyramine, and alcohol withdrawal. Factitious self-administration of sympathomimetic amines by patients with psychiatric illness should also be considered under appropriate circumstances. Cases in which catecholamines have been added to 24-hour urine collections have been noted as well, especially in health care workers. In these cases, there is a marked discrepancy between catecholamine and catecholamine metabolite levels. Diencephalic seizures are a very rare cause of intermittent spells with high blood pressure; in these cases, abnormalities on an electroencephalogram may help secure the proper diagnosis.

Calamitous intracranial events such as subarachnoid hemorrhage or posterior fossa tumor may be associated with increased sympathoadrenal (SA) discharge and the corresponding increase in BP and catecholamine levels. In these cases, the patient has suffered an obvious neurologic catastrophe which can be identified as the cause; it should be kept in mind, however, that a pheochromocytoma paroxysm may result in subarachnoid or intracerebral hemorrhage.

Hemorrhage into an unsuspected pheo may cause an **abdominal catastrophe** diagnosed by imaging, or **noncardiac pulmonary edema.** These presentations are frequently associated with hypotension or shock rather than hypertension.

Localization of pheochromocytoma and paraganglioma

The traditional dictum has been that 90% of pheos are intra-adrenal and 10% extra-adrenal. The identification of syndromic pheochromocytoma, however, has led to the recognition that extra-adrenal lesions (paragangliomas) are in fact more common than previously thought (Table 5.8). Most extra-adrenal pheos are located in the abdomen about the aortic plexuses ("organ of Zuckerkandl"), accounting for about three quarters of these cases. Approximately 10% of extra-adrenal pheos occur in the urinary bladder and an additional 10% in the thorax, the latter generally about the paraspinal sympathetic ganglia. Paraganglia in the head and neck region are not uncommon in the PGL syndromes but these very rarely secrete catecholamines. Visceral locations have also been described for pheochromocytoma but these are vanishingly rare.

Imaging techniques

The traditional teaching is that localization procedures are performed only after biochemical confirmation of a pheochromocytoma. Although this remains a solid recommendation, the wide availability of state-of-the-art imaging techniques, principally CT and magnetic resonance imaging (MRI), has resulted in the inappropriate utilization of imaging earlier in the course of a workup, resulting in unnecessary expense and inconvenience. That said, imaging can be useful in excluding pheochromocytoma where the catecholamine analyses are borderline and the symptoms compatible.

The utilization of imaging modalities should be informed by knowledge of the likely locations of pheochromocytomas. Intra-adrenal lesions are well visualized by CT and MRI scanning. CT gives superior spatial resolution; MRI permits distinction of pheos from cortical nodules as pheos appear uniquely hyperdense on T2 weighted images (Figs. 5.7 and 5.8). On CT scanning, image heterogeneity

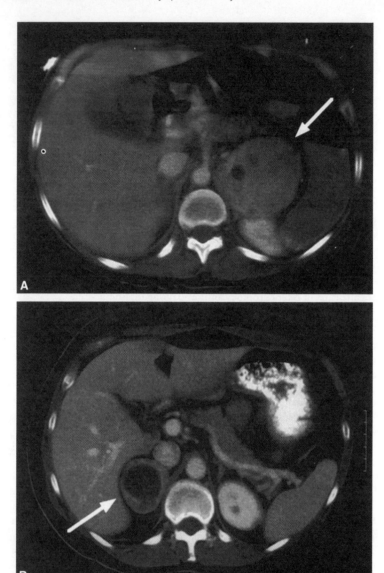

FIGURE 5.7.   A: CT scan of 7.2 cm heterogeneous left adrenal mass. **B:** CT scan of 4 × 4 cm right suprarenal mass with large cystic central component, initially reported as suspicious for metastatic disease (arrows point to the lesions). (From Gillam MP, Landsberg L. *Challenging Cases in Endocrinology*. Totowa, NJ: Humana Press; 2002:155–183.)

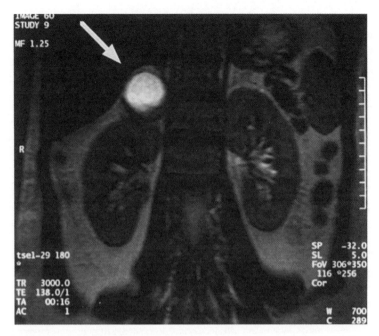

FIGURE 5.8.   MR image of suprarenal mass demonstrated on CT scan with high signal intensity. (From Gillam MP, Landsberg L. *Challenging Cases in Endocrinology*. Totowa, NJ: Humana Press; 2002:155–183.)

reflects hemorrhage and necrosis, common in pheos, with necrotic areas on occasion forming cysts within the otherwise densely solid tumors. MRI is a useful technique for imaging extra-adrenal pheos and for identifying metastases in patients with malignant pheochromocytoma.

Radionuclide scanning with iodine 123 metaiodobenzylguanidine (MIBG), although widely touted in some circles, has a very limited role; it may be useful in localizing extra-adrenal pheos or metastatic lesions when CT and MRI are unrevealing. MIBG is a substrate for the amine uptake transporter found in the SNS and adrenal medulla, and is therefore accumulated in sympathetically derived tissues. The mass of adrenergic tissue, however, needs to be sufficiently great to give an external scintiscan so that sympathetic nerve endings and normal adrenal medulla do not give a positive result. CT/positron emission tomography (PET) scanning with fludeoxyglucose has also demonstrated usefulness in identifying extra-adrenal and metastatic pheos. Scanning with labeled somatostatin receptor analogs has a very limited use when all other methods have failed.

As pheos are very vascular, tumors they can be well demonstrated by arteriography. Before CT and MRI, this was a major way of visualizing pheochromocytoma, but has been rendered obsolete by the techniques described above. It is sometimes undertaken, nonetheless, in the futile (and ill-advised) attempt to demonstrate a tumor when all else has failed. As radiographic contrast media delivered via the arterial circulation may provoke a serious paroxysm, adrenergic blockade is essential before undertaking such a study.

Treatment of pheochromocytoma: preoperative management

The goal of treatment is the safe surgical resection of the tumor. The key to safe surgery is preoperative preparation and skilled intraoperative management. Once the diagnosis is established, α-adrenergic blockade is initiated. Phenoxybenzamine is the time-honored agent because it induces a noncompetitive blockade of long duration. The action of phenoxybenzamine is cumulative, so the final dose must be attained gradually. A starting dose of 10 mg every 12 hours is reasonable with titration up to control the blood pressure and abolish the paroxysms, balancing these effects with the orthostatic hypotension that always occurs with α-blockade. Most patients require between 40 and 80 mg per day but higher doses are occasionally needed.

Doxazosin is a reasonable alternative if phenoxybenzamine is not available. This induces a selective α_1 competitive blockade that is well tolerated. The α_1 selectivity is associated with less tachycardia, a potential advantage over phenoxybenzamine, as is less postoperative hypotension. The fact that blockade with doxazosin is competitive, however, means that it could be overcome with large surges of catecholamines from the tumor; nonetheless, doxazosin has been successfully used as reported in a number of studies. The dose is titrated up to a maximum of 32 mg per day.

α-Methyl-para-tyrosine (metyrosine), an inhibitor of tyrosine hydroxylase, has been used to decrease catecholamine synthesis in very large tumors, thereby rendering control with adrenergic blocking agents easier. Its toxicity precludes general usefulness, however, and its use is therefore reserved for unresectable or malignant pheochromocytomas

Once α-blockade is initiated, a liberal salt diet is instituted to reverse the volume depletion that is always present because of catecholamine-induced venoconstriction. Volume expansion is a critical component of preoperative management and will partially counteract the orthostatic hypotension that occurs with phenoxybenzamine. Once α-blockade is initiated, treatment with β-blocking agents will be required. Ten milligrams of propranolol three or four times per day is usually sufficient to control the tachycardia, but can be titrated up if needed. β-Blockade is also necessary to prevent or diminish anesthesia-related arrhythmias.

Two weeks of adrenergic blockade is generally required to insure safe surgery. As the appropriate dose of phenoxybenzamine or doxazosin is being established, individual paroxysms can be treated with oral doses of the short acting selective α_1 blocker prazosin or with i.v. phentolamine.

Volume restitution can be accomplished by initiating a high salt diet during the titration of α blockade over the 2-week period prior to surgery.

Anesthesia and surgery

Surgery is best carried out in centers with experience in both the anesthetic management and surgical resection of these tumors. Appropriate management includes careful monitoring during the induction of anesthesia and during the surgical procedure. This can be tailored to the clinical findings in an individual case but always includes continuous BP and central venous pressure monitoring from indwelling arterial and central venous lines, as well as continuous electrocardiographic (EKG) monitoring of heart rate and rhythm. In patients with overt cardiac dysfunction, some centers have utilized intraoperative transesophageal echocardiography to monitor cardiac function.

Although opioids are contraindicated in patients with pheochromocytoma, they can be safely given once adrenergic blockade is in place, and, in fact, have a major role in the induction and maintenance of anesthesia in pheo patients. The risk with opioids is in patients with unsuspected pheos undergoing unrelated general anesthesia and surgery. Induction is followed by inhalation anesthetic agents supplemented by opioids.

Minimally invasive laparoscopic surgery has become the preferred procedure for most intra-adrenal tumors, although very large lesions or those involving the inferior vena cava require an open approach. A small percentage of cases will require conversion of a laparoscopic to an open procedure. Some extra-adrenal pheos in the abdomen may be removed via the laparoscope but most will need an open operation.

Catecholamine release from the pheo may be stimulated during intubation, anesthesia induction, and, most importantly, during manipulation of the tumor; the larger the tumor the greater the risk. The resultant increase in BP may be treated by nitroprusside or phentolamine; the increase in pulse rate or the development of tachyarrhythmias is treated by i.v. infusion of esmolol. Aggressive replacement of fluid losses during the procedure is important; hypotension generally responds better to volume support than to vasopressors. It is important to remove the tumor with the capsule intact to avoid seeding of the peritoneal space. Surgical mortality should be less than 2%.

For intra-adrenal lesions, the traditional dictum has been to remove the entire adrenal gland and not try to "spare the remaining normal adrenal." For sporadic solitary lesions, this is obvious because the remaining normal gland will produce adequate amounts of cortical steroids. In MEN 2 syndromes, adrenal medullary hyperplasia and multiple tumors preclude cortical-sparing procedures in patients with demonstrable bilateral disease. If only unilateral disease is apparent on imaging, the contralateral adrenal should be left in place but a lifetime of monitoring for recurrence on the previously uninvolved side will be required; blood pressure measurements, assessment for symptoms of pheochromocytoma, and measurement of urinary E should be performed at least yearly in these patients. In VHL patients with bilateral disease, cortical-sparing operations are a viable option. Most patients will not need cortical steroids but the recurrence rate is not insignificant (10% to 25% in reported series). In these patients, the risk of recurrence with a more difficult second procedure needs to be balanced against a lifetime of steroid replacement.

After surgery, catecholamine excretion returns to normal by about 2 weeks, representing restoration to normal of catecholamine stores in peripheral sympathetic nerve endings. Twenty-four–hour urinary excretion of catecholamines and metanephrines should be checked after 2 weeks to rule out residual tumor. Annual yearly follow-up is recommended for at least the next several years (some consensus panels recommend 10 years) in sporadic cases and for life in syndromic kindreds. This should include a clinical evaluation (BP, symptoms) and a 24-hour urine for catecholamines and metanephrines.

The 5-year survival rate after surgical removal is over 95% and recurrence rate is generally less than 10% but may be higher in syndromic cases.

Malignant and unresectable pheochromocytoma

The traditional estimate is that about 10% of pheochromocytomas are malignant. As noted above, the risk of malignancy is greater in some of the syndromic pheos, particularly the SDHB mutation. It appears that in general the risk of malignancy is greater in extra-adrenal as compared with adrenal lesions. The only definite evidence that a pheo is malignant is the presence of distant metastases. Histologic features and even local invasiveness do not predict the potential for metastases. Metastases most commonly involve liver, lungs, and bone reflecting hematogenous dissemination. Metastases may be detected by PET/CT, MIBG scanning, somatostatin receptor scanning, or MRI, with PET/CT generally considered the most useful.

The treatment of malignant pheochromocytoma is palliative only and involves chemotherapy, localized radiation particularly for osseous metastases, and in some cases treatment with 131-I MIBG. If scintiscans with 123-I MIBG reveal significant uptake, treatment with the 131-I isotope has occasionally demonstrated a tumoricidal effect with a fall in catecholamine production. Obviously, any ablative therapy should be performed only in patients when adequate adrenergic blockade is in place.

Unresectable tumor may also occur in the absence of metastases. Local invasion involving the inferior vena cava or other vital structures, in patients with high surgical risk, may render complex operations impossible. In patients with unresectable disease or metastatic deposits, control of catecholamine excess with adrenergic blockade and metyrosine can provide substantial symptomatic benefit. The prognosis for patients with malignant pheochromocytoma is not good; the 5-year survival rate is less than 50%, but long-term survival has been noted in some patients.

Pheochromocytoma in pregnancy

Special problems bedevil the recognition and the treatment of pheochromocytoma in pregnant women. Confusion with the much more common preeclampsia frequently delays diagnosis as hypertension is the usual presentation; symptoms that suggest the diagnosis in the nonpregnant patient such as sweating may be erroneously attributed to the pregnancy. The carbohydrate intolerance, for example, is frequently assumed to represent gestational diabetes. The presence of headache, difficult BP control, and wide swings in blood pressure should raise the possibility of a pheo. The presence of a gravid uterus may accentuate hypertension in the supine position, and fetal movement may occasionally provoke a pressor crisis. The diagnosis is established by 24-hour urinary catecholamines and metanephrines. Localization is by MRI (T2 weighted images without gadolinium). Treatment is with adrenergic blockade as in the nonpregnant patient.

The timing of surgical removal is dependent on the stage of pregnancy at the time of diagnosis. Before 25 weeks of gestation, the consensus recommends surgical removal of the pheo, done after adrenergic blockade is in place. Later in the pregnancy, the size of the gravid uterus makes operation difficult, so the recommendation is for medical management until near term with ongoing assessment of fetal viability. Spontaneous vaginal delivery is best avoided because of catecholamine surges which are dangerous even in patients with adrenergic blockade. The recommendation is for cesarean section, delivery of the fetus, and subsequent removal of the pheochromocytoma. Even with the most appropriate regimen, fetal and maternal mortality are increased.

The fetus is protected from the increased catecholamines by placental degradation but the placenta itself is not, leading to placental ischemia, infarction, and an increased incidence of placental abruption with attendant disseminated intravascular coagulation.

Neuroblastoma, Ganglioneuroblastoma, and Ganglioneuroma

Other tumors derived from SNS precursors (Fig. 5.1) occur predominantly in the pediatric population, although they may also, much less commonly, present in adult life. Many of these neoplasms synthesize catecholamines, and assessment of catecholamine production plays an important role in diagnosis.

Neuroblastoma and ganglioneuroblastoma

NB and GNB are usually considered together because their biologic behavior and clinical features are similar. In GNBs, mature ganglion cells constitute 50% or more of the cellular content of the tumor, the remainder being immature neuroblasts. The prognosis may be a little better in GNBs than in NBs.

NB is the most common extracranial solid malignancy of childhood. Derived from primitive neuroblasts of the SNS ganglia, this tumor is characterized by considerable variation in clinical behavior ranging from spontaneous regression to widespread rapidly fatal metastatic disease. In some cases, the tumors spontaneously mature into benign ganglioneuromas. The underlying pathogenesis often involves chromosomal deletions which may result in an overexpression of the protooncogene NMYC.

The tumors are located around sympathetic ganglia and the adrenal, the latter being the site of origin in about 40% of cases. About 25% arise about ganglia in the abdomen and 15% in the paravertebral ganglia of the thorax, often presenting as posterior mediastinal masses. The remainder occur in the cervical and pelvic regions. Almost half the cases occur before the age of 1 year and these have the best prognosis.

These tumors contain the sympathetic neuronal uptake carrier which renders them visible on scintiscan with 123-I MIBG. They also express chromogranin A and contain catecholamine storage granules clearly depicted in electron photomicrographs. Interestingly, despite catecholamine stores in the granules, hypertension and paroxysms are unusual in NB patients, for reasons that are not entirely clear. It is known that NE and DA are metabolized within the tumor so that the end products, vanilmandelic acid and HVA, are present in large quantities in the urine; measurements of these compounds thus play a significant role in diagnosis, as increased excretion of one or both of these metabolites occurs in over 90% of cases. The storage capability of these tumors for catecholamines may be less than in the normal SNS structures accounting for greater formation of metabolites and less release of NE. Nonetheless, the catecholamine content of these tumors is large enough to give a dense MRI image on T2 weighted sequences.

Clinical features of neuroblastoma and ganglioneuroblastoma

NB and GNB typically present as mass lesions in infancy or early childhood. They are frequently metastatic at presentation with spread *via* lymph nodes and bloodstream. Metastases most often involve bone but liver and skin are also common sites of metastatic deposits, the latter often bluish purple in color. Spread to lung and dura also occurs but less commonly. A characteristic finding, although noted in only a minority of patients, is involvement of the orbit with proptosis and purple or black ecchymosis. Vertebral involvement in the cervical region may cause Horner's syndrome, a finding that should initiate a search for NB in infants with this syndrome.

Two paraneoplastic syndromes have been noted with NB: secretion of VIP and an obscure neurologic syndrome (opsoclonus myoclonus). The former leads to watery diarrhea frequently with hypokalemia; the latter is characterized by rapid involuntary eye movements and jerking movements of the extremities and trunk.

Treatment is highly specialized and involves surgery and chemotherapy.

Ganglioneuroma

GN, less common than NB, is also predominantly a pediatric tumor, although the average age of occurrence is older than that of NB (about 7 years). The tumor does occur in adults, but less commonly. The tumor is composed of mature ganglion cells and Schwann cells, and is generally considered benign. It is located predominantly in the sympathetic paravertebral chains, most commonly in the thoracic region, where it presents as a posterior mediastinal mass. Occurrence in the adrenal gland is less common. Approximately one half of these tumors take up MIBG and secrete increased amounts of catecholamines. Those that do produce NE resemble extra-adrenal pheochromocytomas; the evaluation of GNs that come to attention with hypertension and increased production of NE are evaluated and treated like patients with extra-adrenal pheos. These tumors may also ectopically secrete VIP resulting in an intractable diarrheal syndrome that, in a number of cases, has suggested the correct diagnosis.

BIBLIOGRAPHY BY CATEGORY

GENERAL, GUIDELINES & DIAGNOSIS

Daly PA, Landsberg L. Phaeochromocytoma: diagnosis and management. *Baillières Clin Endocrinol Metab.* 1992;6:143–166.

Gillam MP, Landsberg L. Pheochromocytoma. In: Molitch ME, ed. *Contemporary Endocrinology: Challenging Cases in Endocrinology.* Vol. 9. Totowa, NJ: Humana Press; 2002:155–183.

Landsberg L, Young, JB. Pheochromocytoma. In: Kasper DL, Braunwald E, Fauci AS, et al., eds. *Harrison's Principles of Internal Medicine.* 16th ed. New York, NY: McGraw-Hill; 2004.

Lenders JWM, Duh QY, Eisenhofer G, et al. Pheochromocytoma and paraganglioma: an endocrine society clinical practice guideline. *J Clin Endocrinol Metab.* 2014;99:1915–1942.

Manger WM. An overview of pheochromocytoma history, current concepts, vagaries, and diagnostic challenges. *Ann NY Acad Sci.* 2006;1073:1–20.

Manger WM. The protean manifestations of pheochromocytoma. *Horm Metab Res.* 2009;41:658–663.

Plouin PF, Amar, L, Dekkers OM, et al. European Society of Endocrinology Clinical Practice Guideline for long-term follow-up of patients operated on for a phaeochromocytoma or a paraganglioma. *Eur J Endocrinol.* 2016;174:G1–G10.

Sutton MG, Sheps SG, Lie JT. Prevalence of clinically unsuspected pheochromocytoma. Review of a 50-year autopsy series. *Mayo Clin Proc.* 1981;56:354–360.

PATHOLOGY

Ayala-Ramirez M, Palmer JL, Hofmann MC, et al. Bone metastases and skeletal-related events in patients with malignant pheochromocytoma and sympathetic paraganglioma. *J Clin Endocrinol Metab.* 2013;98:1492–1497.

Mackay B, Masse SR, King OY, et al. Diagnosis of neuroblastoma by electron microscopy of bone marrow aspirates. *Pediatrics.* 1975;56:1045–1049.

Shetty PK, Balaiah K, Gnana Prakash S, et al. Ganglioneuroma always a histopathological diagnosis. *Online J Health Allied Sci.* 2010;9:19.

Tischler AS, Kimura N, McNicol AM. Pathology of pheochromocytoma and extra-adrenal paraganglioma. *Ann NY Acad Sci.* 2006;1073:557–570.

DA & EPI

Januszewicz W, Wocial B, Januszewicz A, et al. Dopamine and dopa urinary excretion in patients with pheochromocytoma—diagnostic implications. *Blood Press.* 2001;10:212–216.

Morimoto K, Shibata H, Miyashita K, et al. Atypical paragangliomas responsible for adrenaline-dominant catecholamine secretion due to extopic expression of phenyletha-nolamine-N-methyltransferase. *Endocr Abstr.* 2012; 29:P840.

Van Der Horst-Schrivers ANA, Osinga TE, Kema IP, et al. Dopamine excess in patients with head and neck paragangliomas. *Anticancer Res.* 2010;30:5153–5158.

UNCOMMON PRESENTATION

Berul CI, Milner L, Moriarty KP, et al. An unusual presentation of pheochromocytoma. *J Pediatr.* 1998;133:581.

Campos-Santiago Z, Bird-Caceres JC, Ortiz-Betancourt JM, et al. An unusual presentation of pheochromocytoma. *Crit Care Shock.* 2011;14:46–51.

Gonzalez-Pantaleon AD, Simon B. Nonclassic presentation of pheochromocytoma: diffi-culties in diagnosis and management of the normotensive patient. *Endocr Pract.* 2008;14: 470–473.

Grossman E, Knecht A, Holtzman E, et al. Uncommon presentation of pheochromocytoma: case studies. *J Vasc Dis.* 1985:759–765.

Hamdan A, Hirsch D, Green P, et al. Pheochromocytoma: unusual presentation of a rare disease. *Isr Med Assoc J.* 2002;4:827–828.

Kobal SL, Paran E, Jamali, A, et al. Pheochromocytoma: cyclic attacks of hypertension alternating with hypotension. *Cardiovasc Med.* 2008;5:53–57.

Magalhaes AP, Pastor A, Nùñez A, et al. Ventricular tachycardia as initial presentation of pheochromocytoma. *Rev Esp Cardiol.* 2007;60:449–454.

Park M, Hryniewicz K, Setaro JF. Pheochromocytoma presenting with myocardial infarc-tion, cardiomyopathy, renal failure, pulmonary hemorrhage, and cyclic hypotension: case report and review of unusual presentations of pheochromocytoma. *J Clin Hypertension.* 2009; 11:74–80.

Proye C, Geelhoed GW. Pheochromocytoma: "the impressionist tumor" or unusual pre-sentation of pheochromocytomas. *Acta Chir Aust.* 1993;25:224–227.

Sarveswaran V, Kumar S, Kumar A, et al. A giant cystic pheochromocytoma mimicking liver abscess an unusual presentation—a case report. *Clin Case Rep.* 2015;3:64–68.

ECTOPIC HORMONE SECRETION

Ballav C, Naziat A, Mihai R, et al. Mini-review: pheochromocytomas causing the extopic ACTH syndrome. *Endocrine.* 2012;42:69–73.

Carey M, Galindo RJ, Yuan Z, et al. MON-48: interleukin-6 producing pheochromocy-toma presenting as sepsis. *Endocr Rev.* 2013. doi:10.1590/S1807-59322011001000028.

Ciacciarelli M, Bellini D, Laghi A, et al. IL-6-Producing, Noncatecholamines Secreting Pheo-chromocytoma Presenting as Fever of Unknown Origin. Case Rep Med 2016;2016:3489046.

Cotesta D, Caliumi C, Alò P, et al. High plasma levels of human chromogranin A and adrenomedullin in patients with pheochromocytoma. *Tumori.* 2005;91:53–58.

Drénou B, Le Tulzo Y, Caulet-Maugendre S, et al. Pheochromocytoma and secondary eryth-rocytosis: role of tumour erythropoietin secretion. *Nouv Rev Fr Hematol.* 1995;37:197–199.

Fukumoto S, Matsumoto T, Harada SI, et al. Pheochromocytoma with pyrexia and marked inflammatory signs: a paraneoplastic syndrome with possible relation to interleukin-6 production. *J Clin Endocrinol Metab.* 1991;73:877–881.

Hedley JS, Law S, Phookan S, et al. Pheochromocytoma masquerading as "diabetic keto-acidosis." *J Investig Med High Impact Case Rep*. 2016;4(2):2324709616646128.

Ikuta S, Yasui C, Kawanaka M, et al. Watery diarrhea, hypokalemia and achlorhydria syndrome due to an adrenal pheochromocytoma. *World J Gastroenterol*. 2007;13:4649–4652.

Kitamura K, Kangawa K, Kawamoto M, et al. Adrenomedullin: a novel hypotensive peptide isolated from human pheochromocytoma. *Biochem Biophys Res Commun*. 1993;192:553–560.

Minetto M, Dovio A, Ventura M, et al. Interleukin-6 producing pheochromocytoma presenting with acute inflammatory syndrome. *J Endocrinol Invest*. 2003;26:453–457.

Mune T, Katakami H, Kato Y, et al. Production and secretion of parathyroid hormone-related protein in pheochromocytoma: part of an alpha-adrenergic mechanism. *J Clin Endocrinol Metab*. 1993;76:757–762.

Radhi S, Nugent K, Alalawi R. Pheochromocytoma presenting as systemic inflammatory response syndrome and lactic acidosis. *ICU Dir*. 2010;1(5):257–260.

Shimosawa T, Shibagaki Y, Ishibashi K, et al. Adrenomedullin, an endogenous peptide, counteracts cardiovascular damage. *Circulation*. 2002;105:106–111.

Spark RF, Connolly PB, Gluckin DS, et al. ACTH secretion from a functioning pheochromocytoma. *N Engl J Med*. 1979;301:416–418.

Swift PGF, Bloom SR, Harris F. Watery Diarrhoea and ganglioneuroma with secretion of vasoactive intestinal peptide. *Arch Dis Child*. 1975;50:896–899.

Waldman TA, Bradley JE. Polycythemia secondary to a pheochromocytoma with production of an erythropoiesis stimulating factor by the tumor. *Exp Biol Med*. 1961;108:425–427.

Yarman S, Soyluk O, Altunoglu E, et al. Interleukin-6-producing pheochromocytoma presenting with fever of unknown origin. *Clinics (Sau Paulo)*. 2011;66:1843–1846.

Zeng ZP, Liu DM, Li HZ, et al. Expression and effect of adrenomedullin in pheochromocytoma. *Ann NY Acad Sci*. 2006;1073:270–276.

PHEO & INCIDENTALOMA

Nieman LK. Approach to the patient with an adrenal incidentaloma. *J Clin Endocrinol Metab*. 2010;95:4106–4113.

Young WF Jr. The incidentally discovered adrenal mass. *N Engl J Med*. 2007;356:601–610.

URINARY BLADDER

Beilan JA, Lawton A, Hajdenberg J, et al. Pheochromocytoma of the urinary bladder: a systematic review of the contemporary literature. *BMC Urol*. 2013;13:22.

Purandare NC, Sanghvi DA, Jhambekar NA. Pheochromocytoma of the urinary bladder. *J Ultrasound Med*. 2005;24:881–883.

Rosenberg LM. Pheochromocytoma of the urinary bladder report of a case. *N Engl J Med*. 1957;257:1212–1215.

THERMOGENESIS

Petrák O, Haluzíková D, Kaválková P, et al. Changes in energy metabolism in pheochromocytoma. *J Clin Endocrinol Metabol*. 2013;98:1651–1658.

SYNDROMES—PHEOS, PARAGANGLIOMAS

Benn DE, Gimenez-Roqueplo AP, Reilly JR, et al. Clinical presentation and penetrance of pheochromocytoma/paraganglioma syndromes. *J Clin Endocrinol Metabol*. 2006;91:827–836.

Gill AJ, Benn DE, Chou A, et al. Immunohistochemistry for SDHB triages genetic testing of SDHB, SDHC, and SDHD in paraganglioma-pheochromocytoma syndromes. *Hum Pathol.* 2010;41:805–814.

Kirmani S, Young WF. Hereditary Paraganglioma-Pheochromocytoma Syndromes. In: Pagon RA, Adam MP, Ardinger HH, eds. *Gene Reviews*. Seattle, WA: University of Washington, Seattlle; 2008.

Lonergan GJ, Schwab CM, Suarez ES, et al. Neuroblastoma, ganglioneuroblastoma, and ganglioneuroma: radiologic-pathologic correlation. *Radiographics.* 2002:22(4):911–934.

Opotowsky AR, Moko LE, Ginns J, et al. Pheochromocytoma and paraganglioma in cyanotic congenital heart disease. *J Clin Endocrinol Metab.* 2015;100:1325–1334.

Welander J, Söderkvist P, Gimm O. Genetics and clinical characteristics of hereditary pheochromocytomas and paragangliomas. *Endocr Relat Cancer.* 2011;18.R253–R276.

PHEO AND PREGNANCY

Ismail NAM, Rahman RA, Wahab NA, et al. Pheochromocytoma and pregnancy: a difficult and dangerous ordeal. *Malays J Med Sci.* 2012;19:65–68.

Oliva R, Angelos P, Kaplan E, et al. Pheochromocytoma in pregnancy a case series and review. *Hypertension.* 2010;55:600–606.

Pardo dos Santos DR, Barbisan CC, Marcellini C, et al. Pheochromocytoma and pregnancy: a case report and review. *J Bras Nefrol.* 2015;37(4):496–500.

ADVERSE DRUG REACTION

Aldibbiat A, Ganguri M, Bliss RD, et al. Synacthen induced phaeochromocytoma crisis, an unusual presentation. *Endocr Abstr.* 2015;37:EP1175.

NEUROBLASTOMA and GANGLIONEUROMA

Geoerger B, Hero B, Harms D, et al. Metabolic activity and clinical features of primary ganglioneuromas. *Cancer.* 2001;91:1905–1913.

Hinterberger H, Bartholomew RJ. Catecholamines and their acidic metabolites in urine and in tumour tissue in neuroblastoma, ganglioneuroma and phaeochromocytoma. *Clinica Chimica Acta.* 1969;23:169–175.

Käser H, Bettex M, von Studnitz W. Further observations on the determination of catecholamine metabolites in tumours of sympathetic nervous system. *Arch Dis Childh.* 1964;39:168–171.

Kaye JA, Warhol MJ, Kretschmar C, et al. Neuroblastoma in adults three case reports and a review of the literature. *Cancer.* 1986;58:1149–1157.

Koch CA, Brouwers FM, Rosenblatt K, et al. Adrenal ganglioneuroma in patients presenting with severe hypertension and diarrhea. *Endocr Relat Cancer.* 2003;10:99–107.

LaBrosse EH, Com-Nougué C, Zucker JM, et al. Urinary excretion of 3-methoxy-4-hydroxymandelic acid and 3-methoxy-4-hydroxyphenylacetic acid by 288 patients with neuroblastoma and related neural crest tumors. *Cancer Res.* 1980;40:1995–2001.

LaBrosse EH, Comoy E, Bohuon C, et al. Catecholamine metabolism in neuroblastoma. *J Natl Cancer Inst.* 1976;57:633–638.

Laug WE, Siegel SE, Shaw KNF, et al. Initial urinary catecholamine metabolite concentrations and prognosis in neuroblastoma. *Pediatrics.* 1978;62:77–83.

Monsaingeon M, Perel Y, Simonnet G, et al. Comparative values of catecholamines and metabolites for the diagnosis of neuroblastoma. *Eur J Pediatr*. 2003;162:397–402.

Sourkes TL, Denton RL, Murphy GF, et al. The excretion of dihydroxyphenylalanine, dopamine, and dihydroxyphenylacetic acid in neuroblastoma. *Pediatrics*. 1963;31;660–668.

von Studnitz W, Käser H, Sjoerdsma A. Spectrum of catechol amine biochemistry in patients with neuroblastoma. *N Engl J Med*. 1963;269:232–235.

Williams CM, Greer M. Homovanillic acid and vanilmandelic acid in diagnosis of neuroblastoma. *JAMA*. 1963;183:836–840.

Index

Note: Page numbers followed by *f* and *t* indicate material in figures and tables respectively.